Foreign Accent Management

Foreign Accent Management

Mythri Srinivasan Menon

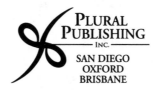

PLURAL
PUBLISHING
INC.

SAN DIEGO
OXFORD
BRISBANE

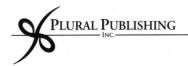

5521 Ruffin Road
San Diego, CA 92123

e-mail: info@pluralpublishing.com
Web site: http://www.pluralpublishing.com

49 Bath Street
Abingdon, Oxfordshire OX14 1EA
United Kingdom

Typeset in 11/14 Stone Informal by Flanagan's Publishing Services, Inc.
Printed in the United States of America by McNaughton and Gunn

Library of Congress Cataloging-in-Publication Data;

Menon, Mythri Srinivasan.
  Foreign accent management / Mythri Srinivasan Menon.
     p. ; cm.
  Includes bibliographical references and index.
  ISBN-13: 978-1-59756-068-9 (softcover)
  ISBN-10: 1-59756-068-5 (softcover)
  1. English language--Textbooks for foreign speakers. 2. English language--Accents and accentuation. 3. English language--Pronunciation by foreign speakers--Problems, exercises, etc. 4. English language--Spoken English--Problems, exercises, etc. 5. Oral communication--Problems, exercises, etc. 6. English language--Phonetics--Problems, exercises, etc.
  I. Title.
  PE1128.M417 2006
  428.2'4--dc22
                                              2006031943

Contents

Acknowledgments

Thanks to all of the researchers and authors in the fields of phonetics and speech-language pathology, as well as my professors, whose work provided me with excellent material for this book. I have drawn extensively from the insights of these experts in determining both the scope and the subject matter of the ideas presented in the book. I am humbled by and indebted to all those whose creative ideas I have adapted in my own practice of foreign accent management.

I thank Mr. Robert Benedetto, President of Creative Arts Studio for lending his voice for the audio portion of this book. I appreciate his patience and invaluable help in the making of the CD.

I also am grateful to my family, friends, and colleagues—who served as my teachers, at home, in school, and on the job—for their numerous constructive criticisms, critical readings, and useful suggestions that helped shape the manuscript for this book. They continue to inspire me in this eternal circle of learning.

I am grateful to my husband, Anil, for his critique, patience, and support. It was he who started the fire of writing and fanned the flames of persistence toward its completion.

And it was my daughter, Sanjna, only a year old when I began the writing project that led to this book, whose delight in acquiring new speech sounds oblivious to my foreign accent struggles inspired my thirst for learning about the subject matter.

And most importantly, thanks to my clients, my students, who asked and continue to ask all the right questions. They are truly my best teachers, who stimulate my thinking about their issues as ideas for all those who aspire to learn English as a second language, to develop techniques and explanations for daily practice.

Preface:
An Immigrant's Perspective

You may have heard comments such as "She is trying to put on an accent!"—or even made such comments yourself. (I admit to being guilty on both counts!) The speech of "foreigners" attempting to reproduce the accent of a native speaker may sound unnatural or "forced" without the use of various linguistic subtleties. Nevertheless, we've all known people who have an innate ability to imitate all accents easily and fluently, often with amusing results. Professionals in the entertainment industry may work very hard to perfect specific accents necessary for their roles. Some people with accented speech, whether a distinctive dialect such as the well-recognized Brooklyn accent or a "second language," have not found the need for accent modification in any form but nevertheless have gone on to achieve success in their chosen careers. But sometimes, for various reasons, second language speakers—like us—decide that modification of their non-native accent is necessary.

The material for *Foreign Accent Management* comes from a place very close to the heart. The birth of this book resulted from my personal experience as an immigrant from India. Like many foreigners, at first I had numerous encounters of the accented kind. Some were funny, a few were embarrassing, and several involved unpleasant stereotyping, but most were educational in one way or another. Because I worked in the field of speech-language pathology, however, such encounters began to falsely raise the question of professional inadequacy. In defense, I embarked on a self-education course to manage my accent, starting in graduate school and continuing into the workplace, with rigorous practice aimed at eliminating my Indian accent.

Practice began with the assistance of my classmates, who critiqued my vocabulary and corrected my pronunciation of words required for school projects. As some of us started to socialize together after class, speech correction continued during "happy hour." Interviewing for a job brought complexities of etiquette and body language to the forefront, along with accent. So my program of accent modification also included nonverbal communication and situational vocabulary. New "accent" encounters in professional circumstances indicated the need for me to put in more practice time using a mirror for feedback. I began to see some results. As the clarity of my speech improved, communication became easier and more enjoyable.

Then I reached a milestone in my accent training: An initial phone conversation with a new colleague I hadn't met yet led to a personal encounter a few days later. On seeing me for the first time, my colleague did a "double-take." Then she stammered out: "Oh! I thought you were an American—you have no accent!" That was all the evidence I needed to realize that my accent management program really worked.

Of course, most Americans can and will continue to detect subtle differences in my

ix

pronunciation and vocabulary. I am still corrected by friends and those family members who are native American English speakers; I realize that such feedback is one of the ways for me to stay on track. With persistent practice, I have improved and managed my accent—but not erased it.

Accent management is hard work—but success is possible. How long will it take? Many years, because it's a lifelong learning process. Your results will depend on your level of patience, motivation, and dedication to practice. But your efforts *will* pay off.

Foreign Accent Management is in essence a record of my personal success in conquering my accent demons, and a chance to share my efforts with you. It's my hope that the techniques and strategies presented throughout the book can help you to achieve success in your own foreign accent management program.

Introduction

As a student of English as a second language (ESL), you probably have read similar books on accent improvement or used CDs and other professional products aimed at accent modification. All of us ESL learners are searching for that one resource or technique for correcting pronunciation to eliminate our accent and reduce our frustration. As a speech therapist, I have observed frustration turning into failure—or into a challenge to aggressively pursue accent improvement. Some people, of course, have a flair for languages and accents—they make speaking multiple languages in the "correct" accent seem effortless. (I used to be intimidated by the ability and skill of such "accent artists." But then I realized we need such people to inspire and motivate us.)

Although the subject matter necessarily includes a certain amount of technical and scientific terminology and concepts (from the field of speech-language pathology), the overall reader-friendly tone makes it accessible to anyone who is interested in learning more about foreign accent management. Simple definitions of more technical terms are provided when needed, as well as practical explanations of strategies and techniques to supply rationales and to promote incorporation of these skills into everyday practice.

This book begins with a simple discussion of communication and its relationship to accents. (Other aspects of communication, such as style, personality, and so on, are beyond the scope of the book.) The focus is on the different areas in interpersonal communication that affect pronunciation and accent and that are influenced by the subtleties of culture.

Throughout the chapters, the technical aspects of speech-language pathology used to manage and modify accents are interwoven with sociocultural aspects of language. This close relationship is a central premise of the approach to accent modification presented in this book. An understanding of speech and language acquisition by speakers all over the world helps to elucidate what an enormous challenge accent correction can be. Correcting pronunciation means retraining the mouth and related structures in different movements and maneuvers, so a chapter on the "speaking apparatus"—the articulators—also is included. Other aspects of speech and language—auditory discrimination, intonation, body language, conversational etiquette, and so on—that influence your accented speech are important for overall presentation of the message and therefore also are addressed.

Principles and Prerequisites

The approach to accent modification presented in this book is based on certain principles, summarized next, along with the prerequisites for success in foreign accent management using this approach.

- This book is intended to be used by persons who wish to correct accents and pronunciation. Therefore, a *good command of the English language* is essential for the student to be able to understand the subject descriptions, recognize the idiosyncrasies of English, and comprehend certain instructions.

- The "standard style" of English is used throughout. Every attempt has been made to present the subject matter in simple terms and to describe techniques so that they are easy to master and to put into practice.

- Speech-language pathology or other technical terms are defined when they are introduced and then used throughout the book. Refer to the Glossary for explanation of any unfamiliar terms.

- The book provides definitions of oral or verbal language and tips on how to pronounce English speech sounds, with sample lessons. However, this is *not* ESL tutorial material that addresses vocabulary building and grammatical structures (English language systems).

- The topics selected for each chapter are based on the premise that a background in specific knowledge is necessary before proceeding to the next aspect of accent modification. Thus, information on accents and dialects, differences between language and speech, the various components of language such as articulation using the oral-motor structures, and how speech sound production affects accents is included as relevant and is presented in a logical sequence for building a framework for learning and practice.

- *This book does not claim that all of the recommended techniques are original.* Some techniques have been in practice in one form or another for many years. It is a compilation that blends valuable techniques with practical ideas that have been gathered during my own participation in workshops, tutoring, and speech therapy, as well as personal experience.

- In Chapters 1 through 12, the instructional text is supported by numerous examples and sample exercises. These features allow systematic practice to reinforce learning of theory and the specifics of language, speech, and accents before the student becomes immersed in speech drills. At the end of every chapter, worksheets present such drills and other exercises aimed at improving spoken English using the relevant skills and techniques.

- This book also offers an introduction to linguistic terminology and phonetic script. This knowledge will serve as a background for learning in the process of accent modification and for recognition of the inconsistencies of language that give English its flair.

- Throughout the book, vowels and consonants are referred to as speech sounds, rather than as alphabetic symbols or letters. Phonetic script—the International Phonetic Alphabet (IPA)—is used to identify the speech sounds and is outlined in the vowel and consonant legends. Those sounds that have spelling variations also are included in the legends. IPA is used throughout the book, especially in Chapters 4, 5, 6, and 11, and in various examples.

- **Note:** Phonetic transcription is an integral part of the approach presented in this book and is fundamental to success in accent correction. Use the tables of vowel and consonant legends provided for practicing phonetic transcription.

Perspective on Progress

- The length of time it will take for enhancement of your English accent (versus *erasing* your native language accent!) to achieve speech clarity will depend on your practice time and motivation to succeed. Success in practice is defined by the ability to detect a speech sound error or other language error, diagnose it, and apply an effective correction strategy.

- The key to accent improvement and management is to follow the strategies and techniques of error sound correction presented in this book. Once you have figured out how to manipulate your articulators using these indispensable techniques, you can "switch" between accents. This gives you the ability to "put on" either your original second language accent or your American English accent—or any other accent, for that matter! American English encompasses a multitude of idioms, often with a humorous flavor. Humor can be a good way to distract a listener from focusing on your accent. It will give you the confidence to control and manage your accent without being embarrassed.

- An evaluation by a speech-language professional may be very beneficial for ESL learners who wish to identify specific undesirable speech patterns. This knowledge can be put to good use in a self-directed foreign accent management program, for optimal results.

*I dedicate this work to Yoga—a wonderful, uplifting practice
that sustains and guides me through the walk of life.*

1

Communication: He Said, She Said, and Finally They Said!

Although accent is the main theme of this book, let's begin by considering what communication is really all about. Communicating is something we all do in our daily personal and business lives. Any place where people meet other people, communication—conveying information—happens. Somehow we have managed to hone this skill of communication and get our message across quite successfully in many different languages and diverse accents. This chapter presents some basic concepts of communication and introduces the building blocks of accent management.

We all have been communicating since infancy in our native language. Because we are well versed in this language, we do not really wonder or worry if the message is getting across. It is different, with speakers of any second language—in this case, English. Initially, every interaction in English can be stressful. Each encounter requires every bit of the non-native speaker's preparation and practice. And if the interaction is not successful, frustration and disappointment may result, so that it becomes difficult to look forward to the next interaction.

Communication or Accent Mishaps

Isn't your accent already perfect—in your native language? Of course it is. But as second language speakers, most of us remember our first communication "blooper" in English. Perhaps we used the wrong word, or our native accent made the English word sound "weird" or different. Such miscommunications are embarrassing—and frustrating too, because as members of human society we want to be able to communicate our message clearly—we want others to really "hear" what we have to say.

Especially if you have repeatedly committed such accent bloopers, you just want to forget the mishap and move on. Unfortunately this may not always be possible—sometimes colleagues may think it is funny to retell the story for laughs while you are squirming, red in the face and feeling somewhat angry. To try to "fix" your initial error, you may repeat the communication attempt in several subsequent interactions, yet still fail to correct the problem. At that point you may take a vow that you are going to "work on your accent" and show everyone what an excellent communicator you are! You may even decide it is time to approach a professional speech-language pathologist about improving your accent. Or, on the other hand, you may decide it is too much bother and develop a negative attitude that may be detrimental to your performance, both professional and social. Whatever your personal history has been, we all can agree that dealing with such accent mishaps is not easy.

Let's look at how you may have dealt with these problems. What did you do to work on your accent or to just communicate better? Currently the market is flooded with tapes and CDs and other presentations from communication professionals who specialize in erasing people's accents. "Erase" is a pretty strong word, especially when used with accents, because getting rid of any accent is not easy.

It takes many years just to modify, let alone erase, an accent, as I can attest to from personal experience. Fortunately, excellent self-help resources that focus on improving accented speech enough to get the message across clearly are available today. Of course, practice makes perfect—so the level of "perfection" is up to the learner. Years ago, however, such resources were not available. Learners of English as a second language (ESL) had to rely on themselves to figure out ways of improving their accent.

For example, determined ESL learners often made lists of words they had trouble with and repeated the words innumerable times while sitting in front of the television. Some learners created several different lists of this sort—one for work, one for social sit-uations, one for interviewing, and so on. ESL learners also tried watching their colleagues *very* carefully in hopes of imitating the correct modes of speech production. Even though more sophisticated resources are now available, such self-help efforts were not wasted. In fact, I devised these exact same practice methods some years ago and continue to use them, along with a mirror to provide feedback!

Using word lists and careful imitation, although simplistic, continue to be very effective ways to practice. In fact, nowadays practice lists not only are included in commercial accent improvement CDs but are spruced up with professional voices recorded in professional settings as materials for practice. So if you have used these practice methods on your own, congratulate yourself on being way ahead of the game.

How much practice is enough—weeks, months, years? Once you attain a certain level of comfort in speaking English confidently, once you achieve a certain level of fluency, it may seem logical to put in less practice time on those word lists, or to stop staring at co-workers to get the r sound, for example, "just right." When you realize that you are not "stressing out" before each communication interaction, or that you can actually have a good time at a barbecue, or, perhaps most important, when that person who retells your accent blooper stories actually compliments you, you feel that you really have accomplished something. It is natural to ride along on a sense of elation and forget to put in time on the practice couch. That feeling of pride is well deserved—but you cannot eliminate your practice time completely. There is *always* a tendency to revert back to old speech patterns, resulting in accented, unintelligible, native language–influenced English. Although inherently not a bad thing, this tendency does make maintaining the new accent difficult.

Here's another illustration of what continued practice can do for you. For example, what would an American English-speaking director of a large manufacturing company do to address problems with productivity? Possible approaches include analyzing relevant production and personnel data, watching an instructional or inspirational video on effective management or creative thinking, hiring a consultant to get ideas on how to deal with the problem, and so on. What would *you* do if you had a work-related problem in your *own* country, where you are fluent if not an expert in your native language? You too would be finding different ways to deal with the problem using the available experts and resources. The point is that no matter what your position within the company, your years of experience at your job, and your problem-solving skills, you may still need to "tweak" your skills in order to be—and stay—effective.

Similarly, we non-native English speakers—who have a long list of accent bloopers, who worry about how difficult the next interaction will be, who never seem to speak American English perfectly—need constant "tweaking," constant practice to stay on track. There is a big difference between *erasing* your accent and *managing* your accent.

Just as the requirements on the job change with every promotion, the requirements for accent modification change with the kinds of business and social interactions you encounter. So your approach needs to be a well-thought-out program of "foreign accent management," for which you are your own manager. As an "accent manager" you must continually work on improving your accent skills for both professional and social situations. Accent management practices need to be continued lifelong if you want to achieve and maintain a higher level of fluency and comfort in English, or in any second language.

Communication and Language

A current topic of interest among people who deal with communication and language is *adequacy* of communication skills, especially in the workplace. This is because adequacy of communication is directly related to the *language* in which the message is being communicated. The message being conveyed by the speaker has to be in the same language of the listener so that comprehension can occur.

This inadequacy in communication may be increasing in importance because there are many more professionals whose native language is *not* English. These non-native speakers of English may be hesitant to communicate because of "inadequate" vocabulary banks or "imperfect" accents, with the potential for adverse effects on how business is conducted.

Obviously there are many other factors that influence adequacy of communication. Whatever the reasons may be, communication is the key to success in all endeavors ranging from interviewing to performance on the job, no matter what your native language is. You have to be ready to master any language that is the language of communication in your field of interest or performance, because communication does not stop with one encounter. And for successful communication, language must *not* be a barrier.

What Is Communication?

According to Dale Carnegie's philosophy of success, it's essential to start with a deep and determined desire to communicate effectively. Awaken your zeal for self-study and benefit from it—this is his message for those who want to improve their communication skills.

Now let's review what we know about communication in general, how it meshes with culture, both business and social, and how it relates to the ESL learner. Probably you already are familiar with many of the basics of communication, such as conversation, interaction, and exchange of messages.

Let's start with a basic definition: *Communication* is the act of conveying a message from one person to another. Hence, it also is termed *interpersonal communication* (this term is used frequently in the field of speech-language pathology to describe "connected speech," or conversation).

Interpersonal communication can have both positive and negative consequences. For example, communication can:

- begin or end a crisis
- begin or end a marriage or a relationship
- begin or end a professional relationship with a boss or co-worker
- earn or cost a promotion on the job
- get the speaker in or out of trouble

- procure or lose a desired employment position

As ESL learners, each of us surely can recall a situation in which an accent or a communication blooper made a difference in the outcome of an interaction. It may be too late to change that outcome, but now it's possible to identify some specific reasons, to prevent similar communication mishaps in the future.

For communication to be successful, *language* is the key. Language is recognized to include not only vocabulary and grammar but also *how* the speaker's message is presented—specifically, tone of voice and body language. It is this aspect of message delivery that ultimately determines whether communication is successful.

Take a look at the communication circumstances listed in Table 1–1. Each of these circumstances requires its own vocabulary and specific mode of presentation. It's easy to see that vocabulary mastered for one situation may not work in another.

Table 1–1. Communication Circumstances

Business	Social
A job interview	A dinner speech
A business meeting	A candlelight dinner
A teaching assignment	A marriage proposal
A departmental meeting	A cocktail party
A training session	A coffee break
A group discussion	A conversation with a friend
A performance review meeting	A birthday party
A press conference	A parent-child discussion
A negotiation meeting	A religious group meeting
A team project	A family reunion

Although some words and phrases may be common between situations, applying them inappropriately can confuse both the speaker and the listener. For effective and successful communication, therefore, many different sets of vocabulary words are needed. In addition, it's essential to use both an appropriate *manner* of presentation (considered later under Face-to-Face Communication) and the best communication *mode* for the interaction, whether social or business

Modes of Communication

You have the language and its vocabulary. But every day you encounter a wide range of different social situations, business meetings, and so on. How do you get the second language vocabulary you have learned to work for you in various interactions?

For communication to happen, there must be a vehicle—a mode or method of conveying the message. The various modes of communication for conveying messages are:

- sign language
- writing
- talking on the telephone
- e-mail
- face-to-face

Sign language refers to a specialized version of communication for those who are hearing impaired. Further discussion of this language variant is not warranted here, but certain communication components that are part of sign language—body language and gestures—are addressed later in the chapter.

Do you know which of the listed modes of communication is your strongest? To be an effective communicator, you must be reasonably proficient in all modes. Probably, however, you are stronger in one or two com-

munication modes—for example, writing or talking on the phone—than in the others. That is fine so long as the mode you are best in is one that makes you effective in your profession. If it is not, you will have to determine which mode of communication is needed or in fact absolutely essential to your job performance to make you an effective employee and successful communicator.

Face-to-Face Communication

Recall five different situations in which you were *unable* to get your information across clearly. Which mode of communication were you using? At least some of these interactions probably involved *face-to-face* communication. This is the most important mode of communication—it's the one in which you influence decisions and persuade others by presenting your ideas and opinions.

Bert Decker, in his book *The Art of Communicating*, explains the concept of *believability* in communication. According to Decker, believability in face-to-face communication equals successful communication. What he means by believability is the show of excitement and enthusiasm in the voice, with energy and animation of the body reflecting confidence and personal conviction of what is said. In speech-language pathology, the technical terms for these qualities are *intonation* and *body language*. Not only an adequate vocabulary but also a show of energy and emotional engagement in the voice and demeanor are vital for the message to be communicated clearly.

Take a few moments to review the following list of examples. The examples are paired so that it's easy to recognize the different manner of presentation that would be required for each type of occupation, in terms of the message that needs to be communicated.

Importance of Believability: Examples

- A business entrepreneur must effectively sell a proposal or her product.

- A manager must discuss poor performance with an employee.

- A school principal must motivate her staff for a unified front.

- A parent must be confident to speak up at a school board meeting for positive changes in children's programs.

- A governor must avert a crisis before it becomes a disaster.

- A president must convince the people that he is the choice to be re-elected.

You must have the right communication skills for your profession in order to be successful. Just increasing your vocabulary for different situations in the second language is not enough. The key is *what you say* and *how you say it*. In addition, your manner of presentation in the second language is strongly influenced by how you say things in your native language. *Culture* has a major influence on establishing believability in communication. For example, you may have encountered a listener who assumes a less-than-positive meaning for your communicated message and thereby becomes active in creating a stereotype. This takes us right to a consideration of how culture influences communication.

Culture and Communication

The close relationship between culture and communication can be demonstrated by comparing how we greet one another in our native countries. and in the region in which we reside. Not only the language used in greeting but also the gesture of greeting will differ from place to place. This gesture may be a handshake, a hug, a kiss on the cheek, folding the hands at the chest, a wave, or other. The way we greet each other rests solely on native culture. Thus, culture is an essential consideration in a discussion of communication.

Sending and receiving messages, then, is a fundamental part of any culture. The people of any culture depend on various modes of communication for practically every type of exchange. In fact, Edward Hall, the noted interculturist, has asserted that culture *is* communication. That is, because culture is significant to behaviors and communicators; it is hard to tell where one ends and the other takes over. Culture and communication are very deeply entwined —one cannot exist without the other.

Today, in the emerging diversity of U.S. workforces, employees for whom English is a second language often experience unfair or disrespectful treatment because of their foreign accent. You may have encountered such an instance in the workplace when, for example, your response was considered less than acceptable because it was presented in accented speech or in a culturally influenced manner. Perhaps it raised questions about your job performance, or caused your team of colleagues to wonder about your abilities as a professional. Or maybe your co-workers just brushed aside your response altogether, instead of putting in extra effort to understand your suggestion.

It may be easier for some native speakers to ignore a person with an uncomfortable difference such as an accent, or to start an intraoffice rumor of an accent-related stereotype, than to spend few extra minutes in today's busy work environment to accept a message presented in a mode or an accent slightly different from the norm. It also is easy for accusations of discrimination to erupt as a result of frustration and resentment from being ignored. Although this subject is a sensitive one, it needs to be addressed to create a healthy working environment.

In this cross-cultural context, communication becomes a complicated issue. It is impossible to send or convey a message that does not have some cultural content, whether it is in the actual words themselves (language), in the way they are said (intonation), or in the gestures (nonverbal communication or body language) that accompany the message. Even if it were possible to *send* a message without any cultural aspects, it is not possible to *receive* one without its going it through the filter of the receiver's cultural habituation. This means that native speakers of a specific language may not interpret everything you say in that language the way you mean it—and vice versa.

In retrospect, you probably can recall interactions in which you might have come on too strong, been too blunt, or otherwise interfered with the harmony of a situation within your *own* language and culture. Now try to recall interactions with native English-speaking Americans in which their communicated message might have meant other than what you took it to mean at the time. The American style of communication, which is known to be more direct than that in many other cultures, can affect interactions with non-native speakers. It's also important to examine your own stereotypes or negative assumptions about American or other native English speakers.

Now let's look at the situation from a different point of view—that of the English-speaking population. It can be very confusing for English-speaking Americans to try to get important information regarding banking, safety, directions, taxes, stock market, telephone messages, and so on, if it is difficult to understand the speaker. Such repeated unproductive communication interactions naturally will create some annoyance, resulting in frustration and even breeding intolerance and negative stereotyping.

Although such frustration and annoyance are understandable, intolerance and derogatory attitudes are not acceptable and certainly not conducive to effective, productive communication. Sometimes an employee or even a friend who speaks accented English is judged as being disinterested in adapting to the host culture; a further false assumption may be that the employee is unqualified for the job. So it's imperative that we ESL speakers make a real effort to better our communication skills, so that the message to be conveyed is done so clearly and effectively, even if trace regional accents are detected in the process. Everyone involved in the communication exchange deserves respect, native and non-native language speakers alike.

What about imitating different accents? My 6-year-old daughter began to imitate her parents' accents at home. I explained to her that it hurt my feelings when she did that. I also asked her how she would feel if we teased her about her "Americanized" pronunciations in speaking a language of India. She admitted she wouldn't like it.

But her next question surprised me. She had heard a few adults imitate her parents' accents and noticed that we laughed good-naturedly. Now she wondered how those adults could get away with doing that while she received a reprimand. Her recognition of this inconsistency raises a good point: By failing to protest when someone imitates a non-native speaker's accent, perhaps we are encouraging that person—who may even be unaware of the discomfort such imitation causes—to continue the hurtful behavior. Such delicate situations are embarrassing and difficult to handle.

Imitating accents to suit a part in the school play may be commendable, whereas imitating to mock can be disrespectful. Some ESL speakers choose to ignore the mockery, on the premise that there are more important issues to fight for. Perhaps using humor to acknowledge deficits in our own speech before others do may make the situation easier to manage. In any case, there may be no easy solution, and the potential for arguments or hurt feelings remains.

When the culture of communication is considered from both American and "foreign" points of view, it is clear that culture will have a complicating influence on the nature and outcome of any interaction. Understanding the negative psychology behind the development of intolerance and the positive psychology behind a successful interaction is essential to break the barriers to communication. Negative psychology such as intolerance may be assumed to be due to repeated nonproductive communication with an accented speaker. Positive psychology may reflect exposure to different American English dialects that are spoken within regions of the United States.

For example, speakers from East (New York), West (California), North (Boston), and South (Louisiana) betray distinct regional differences in accents and vocabulary. Within New York City, in its five boroughs, you can detect Brooklyn or Bronx accents that are fairly distinctive. And characters in the movie *Good Will Hunting* had the well-recognized *South* Boston accent. Although the media comment on, deplore, and compliment various pronunciations and accents, the differences are nevertheless considered acceptable within business and social circles. Perhaps some day Spanish-accented English, Chinese-accented English, or Indian-accented English also will achieve the same acceptable status.

Accent and Communication

Long ago the British playwright George Bernard Shaw (in *Pygmalion*) presented the idea that there could be socio-cultural unity only if everyone in the nation (Great Britain) spoke a Standard English dialect. He was the first to support the teaching of Standard English to all British, in order to unite the culture and stop the acts of social discrimination based on telltale regional dialects. After years of struggle, the different British accents are now considered acceptable within Great Britain.

By this reasoning applied to various "foreign English" accents, should everyone be learning Standard English dialect *and* accent? And if so, which accent (American, British, Australian, and so on) is to be considered the Standard English accent and readily accepted in all facets of communication? Because English or its regional, accented dialect is emerging as the language that seems to connect the world's people in business and pleasure, it probably is being given serious consideration by the members of "who's who in global communication"! A happy result of global adoption of English could be acceptance of Spanish English, Indian English, Chinese English, and so on, as languages of global communication.

So if you are still wondering if accent and communication are intertwined, yes— they are. Although overall, communication depends on *adequacy* of language, accent pertains especially to *clarity* of spoken language. To be understood, use of the right words (*language*) spoken in a suitable voice (*intonation*) and delivered clearly (*intelligibility*) is required. *Accent* is directly related to *intelligibility*.

Despite use of appropriate vocabulary and intonation, the message can still be misunderstood if clarity and intelligibility are compromised by a heavy accent, so that communication is unsuccessful. Accent and pronunciation are critical in all verbal modes of communication, particularly those in which the interaction is not face to face, such as in talking on the telephone or over the intercom.

In face-to-face communication, comprehension may be supported by facial expression and body language consistent with the message conveyed, but these enhancements are lacking in phone conversations. Hence, efforts to maximize intelligibility and clarity by focusing on accent and pronunciation are essential; these are topics of later chapters.

Numerous other factors such as style, personality, and so on will influence the various aspects of communication; however, these topics are beyond the scope of this discussion. Courses to improve public speaking, for conflict resolution, how to be a negotiator, and the like are available; these may be of help to specific ESL learners. But as a quick tip, to check your own style of communication, compare it with that of native speakers; such comparison may highlight some challenges that you need to address. If you can imitate a style to suit your needs and personality, feel free to borrow it. Some ESL speakers are born with confidence and extraordinary communication styles; for such people, focusing only on accent improvement may be sufficient for successful communication. For the rest of us, these qualities can be learned, nurtured, and strengthened through sincere effort and disciplined practice.

Building Blocks of Communication and Accent

Finally, we come to the topic you have been waiting for: How are you going to accomplish successful accent/communication improvement? The primary goal of communication, of course, is to convey your message naturally, fluently, and efficiently, whatever the language. But with a new language in a new country, natural flair is practically unheard of, fluency becomes a chore, and efficiency turns into a challenge.

So what are the requirements for clear, unaccented communication? Where does accent belong within the framework of communication? More specifically, what vocalization and other skills are involved in accent modification? The field of speech-language pathology has the answers to these questions. The researchers in this field have compiled excellent data from work in the area of communication disorders. This body of research and knowledge can be adapted for foreign accent management.

Because modification of accent is the premise of this book, an introduction to the building blocks for accent and communication from the field of speech-language pathology is a logical place to start. These building blocks, listed in Table 1–2, provide a structure and a system to address a problem that has plagued many immigrants for many decades.

All of these aspects of communication are essential to the process of foreign accent management, so a separate chapter is dedicated to each of them (except for style, which is not covered in this book), with worksheets to use in putting theory into practice.

Summary

Now you have become acquainted with some of the essentials in the study of communication and with the building blocks of accent management. The following chapters discuss in detail these building blocks and their significance in accent improvement and communication.

Targeting the articulators (anatomic speech equipment), speech, language, accent, intonation, auditory discrimination, and nonverbal skills is key to making your

Table 1–2. Building Blocks for Accents and Communication

Articulators	anatomic vocalizing equipment: tongue, lips, teeth, throat, voice box, and so on
Speech	sounds that make up words to get the message across
Language	words that make up the message to be conveyed
Accent	distinctive feature of pronunciation influenced by native language
Auditory discrimination	ability to hear critical speech sound differences
Intonation	conveys the message with "feeling"
Nonverbal	communication reflecting the mood of the group or self (body language)
Conversation	exchange of ideas through clear pronunciation
Style	how you say what you say; may be influenced by personality and habits*

*Not discussed in this book.

accent and verbal presentation clear and attractive. Therefore, in addition to providing you with the facts and insights on the subtleties of verbal communication, the remainder of this book is designed to equip you with strategies and techniques to modify your skills in any situation and to manage your accent—not just for a short period of time, but lifelong.

Complete the questionnaire beginning on the following page to establish your baseline and set goals for your program of foreign accent management. You can refer back to it to add data or to monitor your progress.

WORKSHEET 1

Communication and Accent Questionnaire

Instructions

1. Below you will find two lists under the headings of Communication and Accents.

2. You will need a paper and pencil to write down your answers. These answers will serve as a baseline to begin your work on foreign accent management.

3. Try to be as truthful and accurate as possible with your answers. This will help you apply the techniques and strategies appropriately.

Communication

1. What is your native language?

2. How do you rate your communication in your native language? (Can you communicate fluently in your native language in personal, professional, and social situations?)

3. When and how did you learn English?

4. Are you currently pursuing some kind of study of English? If your answer is yes, describe the materials you are using for your study.

5. How frequently do you communicate in English? (hours in a day, week, month)

6. How do you rate your communication in your second language, English? (Good, Average or Bad). Explain.

7. How often do you switch between your native language and your second language?

8. Do you actively participate in meetings at work? If your answer is yes, explain your involvement. If no, list your reasons.

9. Do you actively participate in social conversations? If your answer is yes, describe your level of comfort. If no, list your reasons.

Accent

1. How do you describe your accent?

2. Is your accent interfering with your performance at work? List a few examples.

3. Have you taken any accent improvement courses? If yes, list the materials you used to erase your accent on English.

4. List five words that you are having trouble pronouncing.

5. List five words that you can pronounce clearly (meaning that you don't have to repeat the word to be understood by the listener).

6. Can you tell the difference in your accent between the five words in question 4 versus the words in question 5? (Clarity or accent).

7. Now list five words that you have worked on improving all by yourself. Were you successful? If yes, explain what your strategies were. If no, explain why you think the strategies did not work.

2

Oral-Motor Movements: Lip and Tongue Antics

Now that you've become acquainted with the building blocks of communication and accent management, you're beginning to get an idea of what the process of foreign accent management entails. Because modification of accent is your goal, frequently refer back to the list of building blocks in Chapter One and relate them to your practice, to assess your progress.

This chapter focuses on the first of these building blocks: the articulators, responsible for oral-motor movements. We have seen that effective communication requires messages to be spoken clearly and intelligibly. In turn, the production of clear and intelligible speech requires the right vocal equipment. This equipment is the set of structures and organs called the *articulators*:

- the lips (labial component)
- the tongue (lingual component)
- the nose (nasal component)
- the teeth (dental component)
- the roof of the mouth (palate)
- the throat passage (vocal tract), composed of an upper part

(pharynx) and a lower part, the voice box (larynx), which contains the vocal cords (vocal folds)

- the windpipe (trachea), which channels air from the lungs to vibrate the vocal folds for speech sound production
- the oral cavity, or space within the mouth containing the lips, teeth, and tongue

In this list, the words in parentheses are the technical terms used in speech-language pathology. Familiarize yourself with both sets of terms because although use of technical jargon is avoided in this book, you may encounter such terms in your ancillary reading and references.

The articulators, or vocal organs, coordinate a sequence of movements to produce vocalizations and patterns of speech sounds, called *verbal communication* in the field of speech-language pathology. People who are engaged in this process, however, know it as "talking" or "conversation."

As mentioned earlier, the articulators are responsible for *oral-motor movements*.

Oral refers to the parts of the mouth and upper parts of the throat. *Motor* refers to muscle-directed movement of these parts to help shape the speech sounds. So oral-motor movements are simply the workings of the vocal equipment—the use of the articulators.

Have you ever thought of your mouth and its structures as speech-producing equipment? The word "equipment" sounds uncomfortably machine-like—but your articulators are in fact the "tools" of speech production. In your native language, you are an expert in the use of these tools—your speech is clear and probably almost perfect. It's only now, when you are learning a second language that an appreciation of your articulators as speech production equipment, and of your skill in their use for new and different speech sounds, begins to matter.

Let's review some of the functions and properties of articulators to understand the importance of oral-motor movements for speech production in any language. Here are a few facts about the movement of articulators:

- Articulators are either made up of muscle or directly controlled by muscle.
- Articulator muscles have to be flexible and capable of precise movements to produce the correct speech sounds within any language.
- Articulator movements must occur in a specific manner, in a certain sequence, and at an optimal rate for the production of appropriate connected speech or conversation.
- Articulators have to be anatomically normal.

If any of the articulators are structurally damaged or missing, speech production will be noticeably affected, thereby impairing overall clarity and communication in any language. The first step in addressing the problem is surgical correction or prosthetic replacement by medical professionals. Once this aspect of treatment has been completed, the rehabilitation team, specifically the speech-language pathologist, takes over to address the impaired speech production.

Impaired speech, also termed *articulation disorder*, may affect both children and adults. Determination of the presence of an articulation disorder requires detailed testing and analysis by various health care professionals before speech correction can be planned and initiated. The field of study that specializes in speech correction is called *communication disorders*, and a professional with specialized training in this field is referred to as a *speech-language pathologist*.

In some instances, the articulators may be anatomically normal but functionally impaired so that oral-motor movements are abnormal. Such functional impairment can be another cause of disordered speech, as seen in children who are developmentally delayed, for example. The faulty movements can be rectified by speech therapy to return the child's speech to normal within the native language. In adults, however, correction of functional problems can be more challenging.

And a classic example of such an adult —with anatomically normal articulators but faulty oral-motor movements not due to a medical condition—is a person who is speaking a "second," non-native language that is *accented* with native language speech sounds. Often such adults are speakers of English as a second language (ESL) like you and me, who have normal articulators that move adequately to produce appropriate speech in our native language but often not in the "right" way to produce speech in our second language, English, thereby directly affecting our speech. It is the faulty movement of these articulators that influences the intelligibility of speech and signifies the *presence or absence of an accent*. This is explained further in the following paragraphs.

Accent and Oral-Motor Movements

Now that you know the origins of your accent, it is important to observe how your articulators move when you speak in your native language versus in English. It is therefore crucial to remember the following set of properties of articulators:

1. Articulators are *habituated* to speech sound production in the native language.

2. These habituated movements typically are not applicable to speech sound production in a new, second language.

3. Thus, native language articulator movements adversely affect speech sound production in the second language, English, resulting in accented English.

Let's look at a couple of examples. When an American moves the articulators (speaks), you hear an *American English accent*. This accent is accepted as "normal" for persons living in the United States. When an Australian speaks English, you hear an *Australian English accent*—and this is accepted as "normal" in Australia. Both the American and the Australian are speaking English but with different accents, and both accents are accepted as "normal" in their respective countries.

As a second example, when a Spaniard speaks Spanish, you hear a "real" *Spanish accent* that is accepted as "normal" in Spain. However, when a Colombian speaks Spanish, you hear a *Columbian Spanish accent*. This accent is accepted as "normal" in Columbia. The Spaniard and the Columbian are speaking Spanish but with *different* accents (dialects are not considered here). However, both accents are accepted as "normal" in their respective countries.

From these examples we can draw the following two conclusions. Firstly, we can conclude that the articulators that produce both American and Australian English are anatomically normal, but move in different ways to produce two different types of accented English. Similarly, the articulators that produce Spanish words are anatomically normal, but move in different ways while speaking Spanish in two different countries, Spain and Columbia, resulting in two different Spanish accents. (Differences in vocabulary are not considered in this example.)

However, when the person from Spain speaks English, the same "normal" articulators produce movement that is identical in manner, sequence, and rate used in speaking Spanish, which is that person's native language. Thus, the articulators that produce Spanish words also are being used to produce the English words. Therefore, with the oral-motor movements *remaining unchanged*, what you hear is the person speaking English with a Spanish accent. This leads to the second conclusion: To change or improve the speaker's accent, the *oral-motor movements have to be modified*. This will require the speaker to adapt the "normal" articulators to move in different ways to pronounce sounds/words in the second language that are intelligible to the listener.

This process of adapting the articulators to move in different ways is easier said than done. In addition, finding out that your "normal" articulators are not good enough to produce speech in a different language can be frustrating and challenging. Nevertheless, awareness of the need to change the way your articulators move is essential before you can begin your program of foreign accent management.

Your understanding of how the oral-motor musculature affects the underlying articulator movements so that the speech patterns of one language predominate over those of another determines whether professional intervention is necessary in the management of your accent difficulties. If you are someone who has an innate ability to learn new languages, this approach may not be for you. But for some ESL learners, professional intervention may provide the key to progress in accent modification that could not be obtained through self-study.

A professional such as a speech-language pathologist is trained to test your oral-motor skills and, further, to determine the specific differences or errors in articulation that are impeding the clarity of your spoken language. In other words, if your accent is in any way affecting your job performance, you will benefit greatly from a professional assessment. Such an assessment will identify specific error patterns and assist you in modifying the effect of your native accent on English or any other second language.

Oral-Motor Articulation Assessment

This section presents some technical information regarding the articulation assessment. To help pinpoint "different" or "error" articulation patterns that may be contributing to an undesirable accent, you may choose to have an articulation assessment performed by a qualified professional speech-language pathologist. A variety of testing materials are available, but these are not discussed here.

In the professional articulation assessment, the following areas may be tested:

- speech sounds in your native language that are *not* present in English

- speech sounds or alphabetic equivalents that are *new* for you in English

- place (where in the mouth), manner (how), and voicing (involvement of your voice box) of consonants

- production of vowels

- rate of speech production

In addition, the assessment groups different types of errors in speech production within categories such as the following:

- **omission**—elimination of a sound *within* a word, such as tumbled = "tubbled," with /m/ omitted, or at the *end* of the word, such as have = "ha" with the /v/ omitted

- **substitution**—one sound is replaced by another, such as towel = "thowel"

- **assimilation**—sounds are blended, such as handbag = "hambag"

- **prefix** and **suffix deletions**— dropping e, s, ing, and so on

Other assessment components such as linguistic analysis may not be performed and are not addressed at this time.

The oral-motor assessment will help you to recognize faulty speech sounds or errors in pronunciation and to identify similarities with and differences from your native language. Most important, you will learn how these speech sounds affect your speech intelligibility. With this awareness and some intense practice, you will be able to modify and manage your accent effectively.

Oral-Motor Workout

Now that you are aware that articulators are muscles, you may be wondering how to get those muscles to move in a specific way. The answer, of course, is exercise. Most speech therapists refer to these exercises as oral-motor drills.

Oral-motor exercises initially were developed to strengthen oral muscles that had been affected by injury or stroke or another pathologic condition. However, the same exercises—with a few variations, of course—can be utilized in accent modification training to teach the muscles to move in various ways that may be unfamiliar to a non-native speaker.

Initially, the exercises target muscles of all articulators for general strengthening and flexibility. As error sounds are identified, these exercises become more specialized. For each of the error sounds, they address the different points of placement of the articulators within the mouth (oral cavity) using visual (mirror) or tactile (touch) feedback.

Are you ready to try some of the oral-motor exercises presented in the worksheet at the end of this chapter? The worksheet includes the following exercises:

- Lip exercises
- Tongue exercises
- Jaw exercises
- Voicing exercises
- Relaxation exercises
- Paired speech sounds

Each of the exercises addresses a specific movement with or without the use of a speech sound (vocalization). As you progress in your program of foreign accent management, you will realize that you are using these movements in your efforts to improve speech intelligibility.

The worksheet instructs you to repeat each exercise five or ten times, but realize that the more sets of practice drills you decide to do, the quicker your muscles will become competent in the new movements. You will need all of this practice, because you won't merely be practicing these exercises in front of a mirror—you will progress from practicing individual speech sounds to words and then to sentences in later chapters.

It's a good idea to keep a record of your days of practice and to track your practice times to stay accountable. The old saying "practice makes perfect" is especially true in accent modification: The more you practice, the more you will notice improvement in how well and how easily you produce the speech sounds, especially in new combinations like those in new vocabulary words.

Muscular Fatigue and Oral-Motor Fitness

Any physical exercise can make you tired, but a higher level of fitness leads to a better, more enjoyable workout at the gym or on the playing field. As with all muscles, articulator muscles can get tired too. Some years ago after my first few days of my first job as a speech therapist, I returned home after work with my cheek muscles really hurting. This was because I had been trying to speak in a different accent—trying to imitate the American accent all day long in order to fit into my professional environment!

Moving the muscles in a different manner—a manner I was not used to—in order to speak a non-native language was what had caused my muscles to ache. I tried a warm compress, which alleviated the problem for one night, but the pain returned by noon the next day. After a few days of this, I was convinced that a different approach was warranted, although I felt pressure to speak in a "good" American accent to fulfill my professional requirements.

Luckily, I discovered by accident that oral-motor exercises could help me do just that—speak in an American accent! A few days later, I conducted a morning speech therapy session that progressed as usual: First, I would demonstrate to the patient how to perform the oral-motor exercises; then I would observe the patient's performance of the exercises. In an afternoon session that day, however, I had to first demonstrate the exercises and then repeat all of the trials along with the patient, who happened to need consistent and constant visual clues to imitate the exercise. I realized that as I performed these exercises with the patient, the fatigue in my cheek muscles subsided and the muscles felt more relaxed.

Subsequently, two hours later I noticed that the *clarity* of my speech had improved. At the end of the day, however, the pain had returned. So I repeated the oral exercises when I got home later that day—after the warm compress, of course! Inspired, I did some quick research and identified a few exercises that helped with speech production. I stuck with my practice; as the muscles became stronger and more flexible, my speech intelligibility in American English improved to an enormous extent.

This connection between oral-motor exercises and accent modification is the principle behind the oral-motor workout. You will find that your "oral-motor fitness" is much improved with consistent practice of the exercises described in this chapter.

Some ESL speakers may not feel the need to continue with these exercises if they have maintained clarity of speech in a "non-native" accent for extended periods of time. But facial exercises have other benefits, such as contributing to a more youthful appearance. So it may well be worthwhile to continue your practice!

The rationale for this approach is that oral-facial movements and word and sentence drills can cause tiredness in the muscles of the mouth, jaw, and forehead. You are moving these articulator muscles constantly in a manner you are *not* used to. You are moving the muscles in a different rate and using different sequence patterns in order to produce words and conversational speech, *not* in your native language but in a second, new language. These efforts can make the muscles tired and weak, causing them to ache just as your body would ache after you did a "cardio" workout for the first time. This ache can be described as *muscular fatigue* (MF).

In aerobic exercise, muscular fatigue does not keep the athlete from returning for another day's workout, and repeated cardio workouts make muscles stronger and the aches disappear. Similarly, with continued oral-motor practice, your muscles will become *familiar* with the prescribed movements. As a result, your articulator muscles get stronger and the fatigue decreases. Stick with your practice.

Benefits of the Oral-Motor Workout

The benefits of the oral-motor workout can be summarized as follows:

- It develops the ability to produce *precise* placement and to correct *errors* in placement of articulators.

- It improves the strength and flexibility of the articulator muscles.

- It enhances the speed and agility of the articulators for connected speech.

- It increases knowledge needed to modify sounds within words and thus to improve accented speech.

- It decreases and prevents oral muscular fatigue due to repeated accent modification drills.

How can you transfer the benefits of these oral-motor exercises to your actual speech or accent management? First, you must complete your workout for the specified muscles. Then you can proceed to work on actual speech sounds. If your articulators are not moving in a manner appropriate to a given speech sound, attempts to produce that speech sound will be difficult. In addition, you must overcome muscular fatigue caused by the oral-motor workout and speech sound drills.

For example, if you speak in Spanish-accented English, you may be omitting final consonants in words such as "have" (ha) or "same" (sa). This may be a common error pattern with native Spanish speakers. In such instances, using a mirror for feedback is very helpful. The speech therapist demonstrates the production of the speech sound /v/ for example, by biting the lower lip; then you are asked to imitate the maneuver to produce the sound. The initial practice of /v/ may be exaggerated to illustrate the importance of producing that final consonant for optimal speech intelligibility.

Similarly, with the speech sound /m/ in the word "same," you can use a mirror to observe the exaggerated closure of both lips

to produce the sound correctly. Once you are able to produce these sounds in single words, you can advance to the next level: practicing in sentences.

Of course, the oral-motor workout is not a quick and easy undertaking. But the exercises are possible for any ESL speaker dedicated to accent management. Lots of practice time in front of a mirror will be required. Once you are comfortable in front of the mirror, you will need to take the initiative and try out your new speech patterns in conversation with family and friends to see if your efforts have paid off! It is easy to revert back to old speech habits. Only practice can help you replace the old habit with a newer and better accent habit.

Summary

Training your articulators to move in new and different ways is a *primary goal* in the process of foreign accent management.

Observing how your articulators move when you speak in your native language versus English is significant to overcoming pronunciation difficulties. By gaining control of *how* to manipulate your articulators, you can control and manage your accent. In this process you may end up erasing your native accent and replacing it with the "new and improved" accent. *Erasing* an accent is not the goal, however; *managing* it is.

Worksheet 2–1 presents exercises geared to "work out" each of the major articulators.

WORKSHEET 2

Oral-Motor Workout

The oral-motor workout is geared toward exercising the lips, tongue, jaws, and cheek muscles.

Instructions

1. Always use a mirror for feedback.

2. Each set of exercises can be repeated in sets of five or ten. However, practicing multiple times during the day to achieve precision may be a good idea.

3. You may begin your practice of foreign accent management with oral-motor exercises before proceeding to the speech drills.

4. You may also do the exercises after your speech drills to relieve your muscles of fatigue.

5. The oral-motor exercises are organized under six headings; lip, tongue, jaw, voicing, relaxation, speech sounds (pairs).

Lip Exercises

1. Protrude and then retract the lips while alternately saying ee and then oo, at a slow pace.

2. Repeat Lip Exercise 1 at a faster pace.

3. Place the upper lip over the lower lip. Hold for 5 seconds; then release with a burst of air.

4. Place a piece of paper, napkin, handkerchief, or tongue depressor between the lips and hold tightly (not with your teeth). Do not let go when tugged at. (Resistance exercise for strengthening)

5. Pucker the lips. While keeping them puckered, attempt to move them to the right and then to the left. Repeat.

6. Make exaggerated circulatory chewing movements multiple times.

7. Starting with your lips closed, say /p/ with a puff of air coming out of your lips.

8. Similarly, say /b/, but with no puff of air.

9. Bite your lower lip slightly to say /v/.

10. Round your lips as you begin to say /w/.

Tongue Exercises

1. Point the tongue to make a fine tip. Then relax to make a flat tongue. Repeat.
2. Move the tongue side to side *outside* the mouth, at first slowly and then at a faster pace.
3. Move the tongue side to side *inside* the mouth, at first slowly and then at a faster pace.
4. Place the tongue against the roof of the mouth and make clicking sounds.
5. With the tongue flat in the mouth, pull it back and forth within the mouth.
6. Place a grape in the mouth and try moving the tongue around. (This exercise helps with approximation for /l/ and /n/ sounds.)

Jaw Exercises

1. Open the mouth and move the lower jaw side to side and up and down.
2. Open the mouth slightly and attempt to "spread out" the jaw/lips for a stretch.

Voicing Exercises

1. Place the palm of your hand on your throat. Place the other hand on the instructor's throat, who will voice the sounds along with you.
2. Inhale deeply and release by saying "ah" to feel the vibration.
3. Similarly practice other vowel sounds: /ee/, /oo/, /ay/.
4. Practice voiceless speech sounds: /p/, /k/, /s/, /f/, /t/, and so on.
5. Practice voiced speech sounds: /b/, /g/, /z/, /v/, /d/, and so on.

Relaxation Exercises

1. With the lips relaxed, say all of the vowels, a, e, i, o, and u, quietly, slowly, and without breath effort.
2. Using three fingertips, massage the cheek muscles in an upward motion from the nose outward, starting under the eyes and then moving down to the jaw.
3. Apply a warm compress after long word isolation and sentence drills and practice.

Paired Speech Sounds

1. Practice the following paired speech sounds—/k/ and /g/, /p/ and /b/, /s/ and /z/, /f/ and /v/, and /t/ and /d/—to identify the presence and absence of voicing. (For example, /k/ is voiceless, whereas /g/ is voiced; you will feel the vibration of the voiced sound in your throat. See Voicing Exercise 1.)
2. Continue practicing until you can make the distinction between voicing and no voicing.

3

Language and Speech: Nuts and Bolts

You've been practicing the oral-motor movements you learned in Chapter 2. Now you probably would like to put your newly strengthened articulators to a test. One way is to communicate a message via the mode of speaking. And speaking requires a language—a system of communication.

When you speak using any language, you want to be understood. Misunderstanding and misinterpretation of what is said, however, often top the list of the most common frustrations experienced by speakers of English as a second language (ESL). A common source of such difficulties is the influence of native speech patterns on spoken English. The material presented in this chapter includes a specific approach to address such unwanted effects. Mastery of this subject matter will greatly enhance your efforts at foreign accent management.

This chapter begins with a review of some basic concepts and components of language. Because language and speech coexist, they are discussed together.

Language

Every language has a main vocabulary bank. As regional influences creep in, new words appear, adding to the original vocabulary bank. The English language, for example, starts with a Standard English vocabulary. Regional English vocabulary differences lead to formation of dialects. In addition, slang and idiomatic usages arise over time and in different settings; slang expressions and idioms, which often make up a large part of casual conversation, may be very hard to grasp during a quick exchange.

As you pour over your ESL books, you may sometimes wonder when you can begin to use all that great information to have a conversation devoid of misunderstanding. In other words you probably want to know how language works—how the language that is read between the pages of a book can be unfolded into spoken language or conversation.

Let's start by addressing two areas that are important in the theory of language acquisition: (1) child-like language and (2) native language influences and their impact on learning any new language.

Child-like Language

Have you ever wondered how we as infants and children acquire language? This question has baffled scientists for years, and many a theory has been put forth to answer it. One of the aspects studied is growth and maturity in the acquisition and use of a language.

Scientists have categorized language into child-like language and adult language for their research. The theory is that as a person grows from infant through toddler to youth into adulthood, the acquisition of language progresses through similar stages. This means that the child-like language grows and matures into adult language. This general notion seems to be acceptable to all.

You probably have met an adult whose language was not appropriate for the person's apparent age. Perhaps the reason was evident, such as mental impairment due to a genetic or medical condition. You also may have encountered a normal adult who nevertheless speaks in child-like language.

For example, we all have heard comments such as "Mr. Smith made a childish remark at the meeting." Such comments identify that the vocabulary used in a specific situation was from a child-like language or, in other words, from an immature vocabulary bank. The assumption in the foregoing example is that Mr. Smith is a normal adult and should be using vocabulary appropriate for his age. And in fact language does go through maturation along with age. Because children are like sponges in that they absorb as many languages as they are exposed to, learning a

language from infancy is far easier than learning a language in adulthood.

How does this fact pertain to learning a second language? It means that you do not have the advantage of youth on your side. However, it can be safely assumed that you pass through a child-like language phase to develop adult language skills in whichever new language you are trying to master. Although this phase is short, it does contribute to memorable embarrassing moments and frustrating situations.

To be a successful communicator, instantaneous leaps from child-like vocabulary to adult vocabulary (and back) are essential in acquiring the new language. It is inevitable that learning to communicate in a new language takes time and patience, despite a pressing need to learn the language, especially English, "this instant." Accordingly, knowledge about languages in general, applied to your language may help throw light on the matter of why learning a second language is no easy undertaking!

Native Language Influence

Another important area is that of native language influence. Let's begin with a few definitions. *Native* is defined as belonging to a particular place by birth. *Native language* is the language spoken at the place of birth (or rearing).

For example, if your native language is Spanish, it means you were born and raised in a particular place where Spanish is the language of communication. Dialectical differences within Spanish may be identified if necessary with further discussions in order to pinpoint the exact place of birth. This also may affect how the language is communicated, perceived, and accepted by the listeners.

This discussion of native language is presented solely to point out that *your* native language will directly influence your learning of a new language—in this case, English. You will automatically and unconsciously make sentences in English in the same grammatical way you would in your native language—say, Spanish. Or imagine sharing with a colleague an English joke disguised in Spanish humor. There's a pretty good chance that without the "correct" rhythm and pronunciation in English, the humor will not "translate" well—leaving you staring at the retreating back of your colleague.

Becoming frustrated, you wonder why your English doesn't sound right even though you are using the right words and your vocabulary is terrific. Chances are that your deep-rooted speaking habits are the culprit. Native language influence is so strong that old habits will predominate in your speech unless you substitute other, more effective speech patterns. Awareness of this aspect of language. can decrease frustration and enable more logical and objective practices in learning the new language.

Now we are ready to explore some basics of language itself. As mentioned earlier, the study of speech-language pathology and linguistics covers this subject matter in detail. However, the following section briefly summarizes the general components of and notions about language and speech.

Components of Language

Language is a tool for people to communicate their thoughts into words. It has a symbol structure, with rules that classify the language as a system to be used as a vehicle for communication. Hence, language can be described as having four important components:

- phonemes: speech sounds, scripts or alphabets divided into consonants and vowels

- syntax: (an element of grammar) or word ordering rules
- semantics: vocabulary and word meanings
- pragmatics: use of language for communication

Each of these components must be learned in order to acquire any new language. Although phonemes and pragmatics are discussed in detail, semantics and syntax are beyond the scope of this book.

Because language can be communicated in different ways, these four components of language—phonemes, syntax, semantics, and pragmatics—collectively form language systems. For example, reading and writing are considered to be part of the written language system. Other language systems are spoken language, social language, and professional language.

Language Systems

- **Written language** is reading and writing.
- **Spoken language** is speaking and listening.
- **Social language** is the vocabulary you use in casual conversations.
- **Professional language** refers to business vocabulary used in the workplace.

It is important to remember that language is expressed in different ways according to personality traits—so each of us may be strong in one or more language systems. Moreover, identifying similarities and differences in the scripts, rules, vocabulary, and usage between a native and a second language is of paramount importance, because the two languages influence each other to a great extent.

Learning a New Language

As a second language learner, you already know that learning a new language is not easy. You have to start with a deep and determined desire to communicate effectively. No one can *make* you study a new language.

Once you awaken the zest for this self-study, you are bound to profit from it. Usually you begin by taking many courses to study the different language components of vocabulary, grammar, slang, and so on. Then comes the difficult part of *how* the words read between the pages of a book can be expressed into spoken language. Next comes the test of dealing with the cultural influences within the spoken language; the ability to sound like the native language speaker becomes the challenge. The list seems endless.

For many of us who have immigrated to America, the need to learn English in order to survive in the workplace is so great that the question is not *when* but *how soon* it can be mastered. However, in today's world, learning a foreign language is not just about learning the ABCs within that language.

Learning a foreign language is very likely to mean learning a great deal about the culture, social values, etiquette, educational system, and other socio-cultural concepts and institutions that contribute to the workings of the society in which the new language is used. Although the cultural material requires a lifetime to master, selective readings and self-study courses do increase awareness. Such self-study adds to your cultural vocabulary bank and helps in the communication of daily lifestyle choices and customs.

Road Map to Learning a Language

In the international world of today's global economy, learning a foreign or second language is no longer just an option—rather, it is a necessity. The ability to converse and communicate without the medium of translators is considered a valuable asset. A person who has mastered another language may be *bilingual*—proficient in two different languages—or *multilingual*—proficient in three or more languages.

It is certainly empowering to converse with people from other countries in a language in which all participants are competent—on an "equal footing" in terms of communication. A common language eliminates misinterpretations and paves the way for fruitful interaction. Unquestionably, a common language is a requirement for com-

---

Drowning in Language

Language must be *over*learned. "Once over lightly" is simply not enough. The best way to learn English or any second language is to be immersed in it. This means being surrounded and exposed consistently to that language. Much of language learning is through imitation and practice. Therefore, as a second-language learner, you must persistently speak, listen, and use that language for all purposes, to build confidence to speak the language. When you have mastered the language, your fluency may suggest to your fellow conversationalists that you quickly "picked it up" with little effort. But only *you* will know how deep you had to dive without "drowning" in frustration before you achieved success.

plete mutual understanding and teamwork between any persons, two groups, associations, businesses, and nations.

Given that the world is filled with many languages, the designation of *one* as the preferred medium of communication becomes difficult. Should there be a regional common language—for example, Asian, North American, or European? In any case, tourists and business people alike seem to be choosing English to get their message across. Is English gaining ground as the common global language? The answer to this question is worth thinking about, especially because age and time may not be on our side for learning a new, second language.

When it comes to learning a language, linguistic researchers often refer to language "acquisition" and "acquired" language. *Language acquisition* is the normal process by which innate, inborn, instinctive language is learned. Thus, we learn our native language by absorbing the specifics of semantics, pragmatics, and other language components in a natural, spontaneous, and unconscious way. So learning a native language occurs by means of an unstructured process.

By contrast, *acquired language* is learned, academic, scholarly language. This relates to learning a language through careful, purposeful, systematic study within a controlled environment such as classrooms or educational videos, etc. A "learned" language that is different from your native language is considered an acquired language. This is your goal as a second language learner: to acquire a new language.

Understanding the difference between normal language acquisition and acquired language may provide you with insight on how to approach learning a new language and foreign accent management. And as pointed out earlier, the influence of native language over the new, acquired language must be considered throughout the learning process, to avoid frustration and disappointment.

So how can you acquire and master this new language? Traditionally, learning a new language starts with practicing the alphabet, buying a translation dictionary, and enrolling in a few adult language classes. But what, if any, specific areas of language are being addressed with this general approach? Let's start with a broad breakdown of areas of learning needed for mastery of a new language:

- Build a stockpile of words and concepts (vocabulary).

- Understand what the words in the vocabulary mean (semantics).

- Learn how to organize the words in a sentence to communicate a message (syntax).

- Develop the correct style to communicate the message (pragmatics).

- Understand the rhythm of the language (intonation and syllable/word stress).

- Study body language (nonverbal communication).

- Be aware of slang and idioms.

- Appreciate cultural differences and customs.

- Learn the "correct" accent and pronunciations.

Does what you have been doing so far in your quest for learning a new language come close to the range of topics covered in this list? Take a moment to read over the list a couple of times and relate it to your learning. This may help you to figure out what areas you have been concentrating on and what other areas you should include in your study and practice. Ongoing review of a list such as this (or any other that works for you) can become a system or a pathway for you to use in assessing progress and improving your second language learning.

Because learning areas such as intonation, accent on pronunciation, and nonverbal communication play a major role in foreign accent management, they are discussed in detail in the chapters to come. However, information regarding syntax, semantics, vocabulary building, and so on is available through ESL tutorials or as courses offered through community colleges, because it is not the focus of this book.

Road Blocks to Language Learning and Accent Improvement

Some people have a flair for learning new languages, but for the rest of us, the path to learning English can be challenging. Anything that impedes this learning becomes a roadblock, making it even harder to proceed. For example, time constraints, family commitments, or a demanding job can become an obstacle to learning a new language.

The challenge is not just for those who are attempting to learn English. Many native English speakers who have tried to learn other foreign languages such as Spanish, German, or French also have ended up disappointed by their lack of success. But there are a select few who have immersed themselves in the language (such as English) of their choice and have succeeded.

Besides keeping in mind the strong influence of native language in this process of learning a new language, no single theory has adequately explained why some learners succeed while others fail. Of course, there are a few "foreigners" who have mastered the English language, partly because they may be gifted but mostly because of sincere effort. Most successful learners have achieved their fluency because of hard work and dedicated practice over a significant period of time.

Many native English speakers often express amazement at the linguistic proficiency displayed by some foreigners. "You speak English so well" is a comment that I have heard many a time. They conclude that such fluency is the result of a gift or flair for language learning—or that English must just be an easy language to learn! (We know the answer to that one.)

Now about the roadblocks or obstructions: Have you felt any resistance to learning English? You must have felt some apprehension or even agitation as to why *you* should be learning a new language or culture, while others are not making any effort to learn *yours*. Maybe if they lived in *your* country they would need to or almost be forced learn *your* language. But so long as you are living in a "melting pot" country such as the United States, learning about different cultures becomes imperative; learning a different language, however, is a personal choice.

Still, it's possible to sort out negative or resistant thoughts to figure out what is needed to survive in a new place with a new language. For starters, you need to ask yourself the reason for choosing to live in an English-speaking country such as the United States. And if you need to learn English to communicate in an English-speaking country, isn't it your responsibility to learn it so that you can communicate with the natives?

Of course, the negative thoughts won't just melt away after a cursory consideration of these issues. But it *is* important for you to establish priorities, to generate some positive thought processes regarding why you need to learn English or why you need foreign accent management, instead of drowning in the negatives and creating your own roadblocks.

Some common roadblocks to progress or improvement, as reported by speakers of a second language from various walks of life, have been described as follows:

- Time expenditure: "It takes too long. Why bother?" The length of time it takes to improve English language skills and to learn to speak with an "attractive" accent may not seem worthwhile.

- Time constraints: "I am too busy to go to school—again." The time constraints of career, family, and so on become an obstacle as fatigue becomes a part of the busy-ness.

- Carryover: "I read all the books, but how do I make it work at weekly meeting or at my boss's party?" Most students find it difficult to translate classroom learning to the real world.

- Resistance: "I am doing fine in my job. I have lots of friends who don't really complain about my English/ accent. I don't how this will improve my career or social life." Many are not convinced that improving the accent will be beneficial in all facets of life.

- Influence of native language: "My English sounds like Spanish. I can't make it sound any different." The effect of *native* language patterns on learning a *new* language can impede progress and make the endeavor a frustrating experience. Most students are unaware of this influence and struggle with learning the new language while constantly wondering why their hard work does not produce results.

- Self-consciousness: "I am embarrassed about what people might say listening to my accent/English." Many students demonstrate nervousness, inhibition, and shyness trying to speak in a new language—one they are not comfortable with. When we compare adults and children, the difference

is that a child learning to talk is constantly imitating, improving, and practicing—not paying any attention to the response of others. But adults are nervous and embarrassed to do the same.

Do any of these sound familiar? You definitely are not alone if they do. But the question now is how you can work through these different roadblocks to reach your goal. An old school of thought is "work harder, work longer," for optimal results. This approach certainly has worked for me for foreign accent management, and is one that I highly recommend.

Today's second language learners have far more resources in the form of books, audiotapes, DVDs, and so on, than were available when I started on the path of English accent improvement. The number of teachers teaching ESL courses has definitely increased. Many community colleges and universities offer English language courses of graded difficulty.

In addition, more research is being done, and more books for self-study focusing on developing strategies are being written. Besides those teaching vocabulary and grammar, audio-video products with word models to assist with accent improvement have recently flooded the market. In addition, support groups such as English conversation classes for persons with some knowledge of English vocabulary but needing more conversation practice, have been established at public libraries. Still, the role of motivation to accept the challenge of a new language, the enthusiasm for continued practice, and the incentive to succeed outweighs the available resources.

When I was an ESL student some years ago, my basic resources were my articulation textbook, the television, the radio, and a mirror. Just as important to my success, however, along with a deep-seated desire to erase my accent, were my classmates and colleagues, whom I would recruit to demonstrate the word patterns and accents. They would work with me after school, always demonstrating patience and respect. Some would even follow up with a mock test to make sure my practice paid off. With this one-on-one attention, my progress was much faster than I ever could have achieved on my own.

Language Changes Over Time . . .

With American culture embracing Eastern practices and customs such as yoga, martial arts, and the like, and enjoying a variety of ethnic foods from both East and West, it is no surprise that many words from other languages have become a part of English. Take a peek into a late-edition dictionary—you may notice words like guru, karma, sushi, tortilla, jalapeno, gnocchi, grande, à la mode, and jihad, to mention a few, that did not appear in earlier editions.

The influence of social and cultural variations that have become a habit or the natural fit of foreign words within colloquial usage among people has developed into new vocabulary for that language. The new words with repeated use gain familiarity and become elevated to a level of sophistication. The phrase "melting pot" seems apt: Newcomers find their initial inhibitions to different cultural practices melting away, as their own practices begin to merge with existing customs. For interested readers, the *Oxford Dictionary of Foreign Words and Phrases* covers over 8000 such words and phrases from more than 40 different languages.

Speech: The Act of Speaking

While language deals with forming a vocabulary/thought bank, speech deals with the actual act of putting the thoughts into words so they can be heard.

The act of speaking requires the use of vocal organs—those parts of the body that produce speech. Because vocal organs assist in speech production, they are referred to as *articulators*. Although you already have studied articulators with respect to oral-motor movement (in Chapter Two), the following discussion provides insight on actual speech production.

Articulators

Although the primary function of the vocal organs is to fulfill the basic biological needs of breathing and eating, they also are involved in producing speech. The vocal organs, or articulators, are:

- the lips
- the tongue
- the teeth
- the roof of the mouth or palate
- the vocal tract or throat, composed of the pharynx (upper part) and the larynx or voice box (lower part), which contains the vocal folds
- the nose
- the trachea or windpipe
- the oral cavity—the space created by the mouth (lips, teeth, and tongue)

Articulators also are classified into the following categories.

- *Passive* articulators are those parts of the vocal tract that do not move. They are the upper front teeth (used to produce the /th/ and other sounds), the ridge behind the upper teeth (used for /t/, /s/), and the bony arch behind this ridge called the hard palate (used for /j/ as in the word "you").
- *Active* articulators are those organs that can move under the control of

the speaker. They are the lips, jaw, tongue, upper part of the throat called the pharynx, and the muscular tissue that hangs at the back of the throat called the soft palate, or velum. The movements of these organs vary depending on the speech sound that is being produced. This variation is under the control of the speaker, to form the correct sound.

Technical/medical discussions may describe each organ in terms of muscles, nerves, and blood supply, which is necessary in the field of speech-language pathology. However, that is not within the scope of this book. Still, some explanation is warranted concerning the part the vocal organs play in speech, especially in relation to accents.

Let's begin with the basics. It's obvious that the vocal organs need to move to produce speech. Just as the different parts of the body—arms, legs, neck—are moved by their different muscles, each of the vocal organs also is moved by its own muscle or set of muscles. And just as you direct the muscles of your arms and legs to control their movement, you use oral muscles to control and move your vocal organs. The movement produced by the muscles of the vocal organs creates speech.

Notice that muscle movements typically are under *conscious* control. For example, with a tongue maneuver such as licking the lips, you are fully aware that you are performing the movement. Other tongue movements you use every day, such as in chewing or swallowing, may be *unconscious*.

Most people are not aware of how they use their vocal organs to produce the sounds of speech, because like tongue movements used in chewing or swallowing, the vocal organ movements used in speaking are performed in a natural, unconscious process. But careful practice can bring awareness of how each speech sound is produced—and

with it the chance to correct some unwanted speech patterns.

Presented next is a short exercise you can perform to discover for yourself how certain speech sounds are produced. Before you proceed, however, familiarize yourself with the terms in the earlier list of articulators, because they are used often throughout the book.

Find yourself a mirror and take a seat. Open your mouth as wide as you can and check out your vocal organs. (Don't worry about cavities and dentist visits right now.) Look in your mouth with a whole new vision—a vision of how these organs that you eat with and brush every day can help you modify your language!

Now move your lips slowly, making the sound /p/ as in /pah/. As you control and operate the vocal organs or articulators in the oral cavity, you are varying the shape of the space that assists in speech sound production. The air from the lungs travels up through the tube and out of the lips to produce the sound /p/. This speech production is also referred to as *articulation*. Following is a technical definition for articulation or speech.

Articulation

Articulation is the production of speech sounds using the air flow from the voice box and manipulation of different vocal organs or articulators. Articulation also is influenced by resonance (sound quality) in cavities (hollow spaces) of the throat (pharyngeal), mouth (oral) and nose (nasal). The ease of articulation is directly related to the flexibility, mobility and precision of the articulators, effortlessness of the air flow, and clarity of the resonance cavities. The words *articulation* and *speech* are used interchangeably throughout the book.

To produce the sound /t/ or /tah/, you involve the teeth and less of the lips. This changes the shape of the oral cavity when compared with that in the production of /p/, and the air coming up from the tube goes through this different-shaped cavity, producing a different sound: /t/.

The different variations in the shape of the oral cavity and vocal tract brought about by the articulators produce diverse speech sounds that are broadly classified as vowels and consonants. The vowels and consonants are discussed in later chapters.

Articulators and World Languages

Every language in the world uses the same set of articulators to produce the speech sounds of that language. However, the variation in the oral motor movements of these articulators is what affects the sound production and distinguishes the difference in pronunciation, leading to different accents such as "accented English" or its variations. Training your articulators to move in a different way—that is, different from the way you move them to speak your native language—is one of the most important phases in the process of accent improvement and is continually addressed throughout the book.

The International Phonetic Alphabet (IPA)

Have you ever wondered if there was one universal language or set of symbols that could be written or spoken and that everyone could understand? There *is* one such set of symbols: the International Phonetic Alphabet (IPA). Here's how it came about.

Written language uses the system of alphabets to create messages. However, language researchers noticed that some of the alphabets had multiple variations in their sound production (for example, the /ch/ in "chaos" is /k/ and the /k/ in "kite" also is /k/). This made it difficult to identify the right pronunciation in written scripts. For this reason, language had to be broken down further into speech sounds, not alphabets, to include the different variations. Consequently, researchers came up with a system of symbols to identify speech sounds and its variations; this was the IPA system.

The first version of the IPA was published in 1888 and may be described as a set of universal letter symbols. It was devised by a group of language teachers in France, who found the practice of phonetics useful in their work and wanted to make the methods widespread. The main idea was use of a separate letter symbol for each distinct sound, with the same symbol for that sound applicable in any language. The IPA has been adapted and modified several times and is widely used in dictionaries and textbooks throughout the world.

But how IPA can help with second language learning or foreign accent management? To answer this question, let's begin by looking at some of the pitfalls in second language learning.

What second language learners do automatically in order to translate or literally "decode" an accent is to fall back on their native language. So if your native language is Chinese, Korean, Arabic, Hindi, or French, or any language other than English, you will tend to use the characters or speech sounds found in that language to decipher an English word. I see this every week in my English conversation class. Dictionaries from numerous languages are whipped out in a flash by the students trying to decipher the new word!

The problem here is that you are assuming that the English speech sound system is *same* as your native speech sound system. You are partially right—there are a few speech sounds that are common to many languages. But there are other speech sounds that may be different or even nonexistent in your native language, or vice versa.

First you have to figure out if there are some sounds in English that are missing in your native language, or that differ from their corresponding native language sounds. Then you will have to develop ways to symbolize those specific sounds in English that are not found in your native language. This is where the IPA system is invaluable. The use of IPA symbols for pronunciation is essential, especially with accents. The best part is that they can be applied to speech sounds in any language.

However, no two languages will automatically have the same *number* or *group* of symbols for speech sounds, because no two spoken languages are alike. Let's consider the languages that I am familiar with from India: Sanskrit, Hindi, and Kannada. Although these languages have sounds that can be symbolized using the IPA, they also have additional sounds that are not found in English. So when I wondered why the listener did not comprehend, it was probably because I used these additional sounds when speaking English.

For example, pronounce the word "pen." In English, the speech sound /p/ is produced with a puff of air coming out—it is called an aspirated sound (in linguistics, aspiration means expelling air) and is pronounced /pah/. By contrast, in my native language, the letter equivalent of p has two sounds, one with and one without aspiration: /p/ and /pah/. Many years ago when I asked a classmate for a pen, I pronounced the word using a /p/ sound, *without* aspiration. Her response was unexpected: "I don't know a Ben." To her, my /p/ sounded like /b/ without the puff of air! In actuality the correct pronunciation in English is /pah en/—a /p/ *with* aspiration.

A person with knowledge of IPA symbols could read aloud an article written in any language, even if he or she did not know that language. This is possible because the basis of International Phonetic Alphabet is that *each speech sound* in any language has only *one symbol*. Therefore, when a word is spelled phonetically, there is only *one* way to pronounce it. This makes the system of IPA invaluable for learning a second language and for foreign accent management.

Phonemes: Speech Sounds

To better understand IPA, a brief introduction to how speech sounds are produced may be necessary. Keep in mind that the terminology of alphabets, scripts, and speech sounds is going to be used interchangeably throughout the book. In the field of speech-language pathology, speech sounds are referred to as phonemes. The phonemes are classified as vowels or consonants.

Vowels (a, e, i, o, u, y and its variants) are phonemes that are produced with no obstruction in the oral cavity. This means that the air flows freely from the lungs and out through the mouth and nose to produce the vowel sound. With the remaining phonemes, the consonants, the air flow is obstructed by the articulators, or vocal organs. That means the air cannot escape without producing audible sounds of friction, because of the degree of closure of the articulators and narrowing of the vocal tract.

Vowel sounds are the most important speech sounds within words that influence a person's accent. It is safe to assume that dedicated practice to master vowel sounds will greatly enhance clarity and speech intelligibility. Hence, a whole chapter is devoted to understanding and learning of vowel sounds. Consonants, on the other hand, are the supportive speech sounds that help complete the vowel patterns to form words. They are discussed further in later chapters.

Let's take a look at how the IPA scripts for phonemes are different from alphabets. Although some of the scripts are same as letters of the alphabet, others are different. It is almost like learning another new script for a new language. But this new script will help you learn any language easily. Refer to Tables 3–1 and 3–2 to study the differences between alphabets and IPA scripts classified as Vowel and Consonant Legends.

The five vowels in the English alphabet—a, e, i, o, and u—can be joined in combinations such as ea in "beat" or oo in "hoofs" to create long or short sounds. These sounds need to have a symbol of their own (a detailed list is included in the chapter five on vowels). As second language learners we try to sound out words as we learn how to spell them in English, only to find out that we are missing letter combinations. Because some English words are

not spelled the way they are pronounced, it becomes hard for second language learners to grasp the language. This is where the IPA system of symbols helps: It provides a

Table 3–2. Consonants in Alphabetic and Phonetic Script

Consonant Legend	
Speech Sound	**IPA**
P	p
B	b
K	k
G	g
Th	θ
Dh	ð
T	t
D	d
S	s
Z	z
Ch	tʃ
Dz	dʒ
Sh	ʃ
Zh	ʒ
M	m
N	n
Ng	ŋ
H	h
L	l
F	f
R	r
V	v
W	w
Ya	j

Table 3–1. Vowels in Alphabetic and Phonetic Script

Vowel Legend	
Speech Sound	**IPA**
e	ɛ
e	e
i	ɪ
i	ɨ
u	ʊ
u	u
u	ju
o	o
o	ɔ
a	a
a	ɑ
a	æ
u	ʌ
a	ə

separate sound symbol for each of these sounds.

Looking at Table 3–1, you may notice that the basic five vowel sounds of the English language can actually have fourteen vowel symbols in the IPA. When the IPA symbol is used, the speaker or the reader does not have to guess how the word is spelled or whether it is pronounced with a long or a short sound. Learning the different IPA vowel symbols will help the ESL speaker to enhance clarity and speech intelligibility greatly.

Now let's take a look at the list of consonant sounds. Eliminating the five vowels, there still twenty-four consonant sounds in the IPA system. Each of the consonant combinations, such as th, ch, or ing, has a symbol all its own!

If you are still wondering how learning of IPA speech sounds can help you eliminate your accent, the answer is easy. To identify the error patterns in your pronunciation, you must think of words in terms of *speech sounds*, rather than spelling. A professional speech-language pathologist will be able to perform an evaluation to assist in this identification process.

Once the error sounds are identified, you can compare them with the speech sounds in your native language and then list the differences. This step is very important to detect the extent of native language influence on the second language or, in this case, your accent in English. Furthermore, identifying the speech sounds using the phonetic script will assist you to keep monitoring your own pronunciation, to promote your best "accent-free" speech.

"But will my native language accent be erased?" you may be wondering. Or can learning the IPA script actually wipe out the native language influences on a new language? You may have received compliments from people such as "You speak so fluently, I can't detect any accent" or "I would never

have guessed you had a Spanish background." But to maintain fluency in this new "accent" requires constant practice and hard work.

Furthermore, at times when emotional currents are running high, you may let go of your new "accent-free" speech and slip back to native language-accented speech. As second language speakers, we tend to "forget" the new accent when we lose our composure during an argument or a disagreement, socially or professionally. (This may happen right in the middle of an important meeting!) Such lapses are perfectly understandable—even if you seem to erase your accent on the surface, you cannot erase who you are deep inside. Once peace returns, however, you will regain the new accent poise that you have worked so hard to master.

Summary

By now you are familiar with the basics of language acquisition and learning and with the concept of alphabets as systems of speech sounds. You know that language and speech cannot function separately.

The key is to remember the effects of native language patterns on learning a new language—in this case, English—during the process of learning a second language. Because native language patterns are old, comfortable habits, they are hard to break. Thorough familiarity with the IPA, coupled with persistent practice using *correct models*, will guide you on this path of accent modification and management.

A few words on English spelling: English spelling is known for its disparities and inconsistencies. This means that the way the words are spelled may not be the way they are pronounced. Hence, representation of vowels and consonants as the sounds of the alphabet using the IPA is an integral part of self-study for foreign accent management.

It has been debated whether spelling and pronunciation should be taught together, especially to ESL students. Because of the variation in spelling patterns that characterizes English, it is considered an *unphonetic* language—words are not always pronounced as they are spelled. Therefore, phonetic forms of the speech sounds (not the alphabet script!) should be utilized to help with the correction of pronunciation errors and accent modification. More information on using phonetic alphabets is presented in Chapter Four.

Worksheets 3–1 and 3–2 present practice exercises for the material covered in this chapter.

WORKSHEET 3–1

Vowels in Alphabetic and Phonetic Script

Instructions:

1. Always use a mirror for feedback.

2. Use the fourth column of the following Vowel Legend table to practice copying the IPA symbols until you become familiar with them.

3. Try to use the symbols in simple words at first, before proceeding to longer and more complex words.

4. As you write each symbol, say the sound out aloud in order for you to hear it correctly when pronounced in a word or when you have to pronounce it in order to correct your accent.

5. Pay particular attention to long and short vowel sounds. (s) stands for short vowels sounds and (l) stands for long vowel sounds. As you say the sounds out aloud, prolong the long vowels—long enough for you to hear the sound clearly. It may seem that you are exaggerating the sound production, but during practice, some exaggeration is acceptable. Once you transfer that sound into words and within a conversation, the sound is adjusted to the pace of conversational speech.

6. Concentrate only on the vowel sounds within the words first. Ignore the consonant sound for this particular practice. For example, say the word /seat/, and then isolate the vowel sound /i/making sure you are prolonging the sound (long vowel). If you make the /i/ sound short the word will change to /sit/ with a short vowel sound.

7. Add your own words for additional practice.

Vowel Legend

Speech Sound	IPA	Example Word	Practice Symbols	Practice Words
e (s)	ɛ	bed		
e (l)	e	able		
i (s)	ɪ	sit		
i (l)	ɨ	seat		
u (s)	ʊ	bull		
u (l)	u	mood		
u (l)	ju	tube		
o (l)	o	goat		
o (s)	ɔ	ball		
a (s)	a	palm		
a (l)	ɑ	fox		
a (s)	æ	had		
u (s)	ʌ	but		
a (s)	ə	about		

WORKSHEET 3–2

Consonants in Alphabetic and Phonetic Script

Instructions:

1. Always use a mirror for feedback.

2. Use the fourth column in the following Consonant Legend table to practice copying the IPA symbols until you become familiar with them.

3. Try to use the symbols in simple words at first, before proceeding to longer and more complex words.

4. As you write the symbols say the sounds out aloud in order for you to hear it correctly. You can begin by saying them in isolation (individually) and then within a word. This will help to learn to monitor yourself when you have to pronounce it in order to correct your accent.

5. Pay particular attention to position of your lips and presence or absence of air expelled out of the mouth. (more information in later chapters)

6. Concentrate only on the consonant sounds for this practice. Ignore the vowel sounds.

7. Add your own words for additional practice.

Consonant Legend

Speech Sound	IPA	Example Word(s)	Practice Symbols	Practice Words
P	p	pat		
B	b	bag		
K	k	kit/cat		
G	g	gum		
Th	θ	thin		
Dh	ð	them		
T	t	ten		
D	d	dim		
S	s	sin/cinema		
Z	z	maze/close		
Ch	tʃ	chap		
J	dʒ	jam/age		
Sh	ʃ	sheep		
Zh	ʒ	Asia		
M	m	map		
N	n	nip		
Ng	ŋ	sing		
H	h	happy		
L	l	lap		
F	f	fan		
R	r	rim		
V	v	van		
W	w	wit		
Ya	j	yam		

4

Phonetic Transcription: The "DNA" of the International Phonetic Alphabet

I hope that the introduction to International Phonetic Alphabet (IPA) in the previous chapter did not throw you into a downward spiral. Instead, I am optimistic that it provided you with the right ammunition to target your foreign accent management with renewed vigor.

This chapter focuses on how to use the IPA phonetic symbols to "spell" words. It has been stated many times that accent differences or pronunciation challenges occur because the spelling in English is *unphonetic* —that is, words are not always pronounced the way they are spelled. If "normal" spelling consistently reflected actual pronunciation, however, use of phonetic symbols such as those of the IPA would not be necessary.

Many researchers and practitioners have debated whether spelling and pronunciation should be taught together, especially to students of English as a second language.

Because of the variation in spelling patterns that makes the English language unphonetic, combined emphasis on spelling and pronunciation may make learning the language slightly easier. However, for courses of study aimed at enhancing clarity of speech by modifying accents, phonetic format of the speech sounds using the IPA *should* be taught, to help learners begin their study on the right track. This will equip them with the tools for correcting their pronunciation errors, with consequent success in accent modification. In my experience, use of IPA script along with word and sentence drills was immensely helpful.

How then do we utilize this wonderful set of IPA symbols for foreign accent management? Let's begin by defining a procedure called phonetic transcription. *Phonetic transcription* is the process of writing words using the phonetic script. In this specialized script, the IPA, each speech sound has a symbol. The process of transcription begins with the identification of the sounds within the words. Each sound is then written using the IPA script.

Let's try phonetic transcription of the word "going." In English, the total number of letters used to spell this word is five. If you listen carefully, however, there are only three distinct speech sounds: /g/, /o/, and /ing/. Hence, using IPA script, it is transcribed or "spelled" /goŋ/—with only three distinct sounds and three symbols.

Because we know that English is unphonetic, meaning not pronounced the way it is spelled, how do we pronounce the words with more than one vowel sound, as in "meat," "suite," "smooth," and so on? Spelling variations as in groups of letters such as ee, ea, oa, ui, oo, and so on, also are represented within the IPA format. Although each of the vowels in these letter combinations ordinarily has its own distinct sound in English, in combination within a word they represent a *single* sound. Hence they are represented as a *single* sound within IPA script.

For example, say the words "meet," "beat," "coat," "suit," and "foot." Critically listen to which of the two vowels within the letter combinations is more prominent in pronunciation—one or both. In the word "meet," although there are two e's, only one e sound is heard. In the word "beat," this single sound is e, not a; in "coat," it is o, not a; and so on. Hence, in IPA format, these sound combinations are denoted with *one* symbol because they have only *one* speech sound. So /meet/ is written as /mɨt/, /beat/ as /bɨt/, /coat/ as /cot/, /suit/ as /sut/, and /foot/ as /fʊt/. Notice that with only one symbol, pronunciation is simplified; you don't have to figure out whether one or both vowels need to be spoken.

Learning phonetic transcription requires both time and dedication, to achieve the necessary level of familiarity with the different symbols—almost as if you were learning *another* new language. There are no shortcuts to learning the symbols: They must be *memorized*. But I can assure you that it is worth every minute of your effort. In addition, drills provided in the worksheet found at the end of this chapter will get you started on the right track. Experiment with this new tool of phonetic transcription. You have to put it into practice so that you can see the results in your speech. Persistent effort will take you to your desired result.

Initially, familiarize yourself with each symbol and its sound in isolation. Then proceed to training your ears to hear (auditory discrimination; see Chapter 8) each of the sounds independently, using the symbols. Gradually you will learn to isolate each sound within a word.

Your study will begin with vowel sounds, because accurate production of vowel sounds is crucial to arrive at the "right" pronunciation of the word. You will learn how vowel sounds are produced in the next chapter, but right now start by simply familiarizing yourself with these sounds.

Importance of Phonetic Transcription

You probably are thinking that you already have a system that you use to transcribe your second language: your native language! That means if your native language is Chinese, Korean, or Hindi, for example, you will tend to use the characters found in that language to decipher the English word.

The problem is that the English speech sound system is not the same as your native sound system. Once you figure out there are some sounds missing, you will have to develop ways to symbolize those specific sounds in English that are not found in your native language. For this purpose, the IPA system is invaluable.

For new language learners, knowledge of phonetic transcription allows retrieval of specific, accurate, and clear information of the word from a dictionary. Different dictionaries use different formats for transcription and pronunciation, so it's in your best interest to find the "right" dictionary—one that uses the IPA format to phonetically transcribe all of the words. *Merriam-Webster's Collegiate Dictionary* uses the IPA format for its phonetics and is highly recommended.

Phonetic transcription demonstration and practice exercises are included after the tables of detailed vowel and consonant legends, presented next.

Vowel and Consonant Legends

Tables 4–1 and 4–2 are charts that correlate the spelling variations in the English language with their IPA phonetic symbols. The most common variations are summarized in these two tables. Other variations (irregular forms) are listed as exceptions in the worksheets throughout this book and may have to be memorized for mastery.

Tables 4–3, 4–4, and 4–5 list the vowels, "r-colored" vowels, and consonants and their IPA counterparts for easy viewing.

Table 4–1. Vowel Legend (Spelling Variations)

Speech Sound	IPA	Vowel Length	Example Word(s)	Speech Sound	IPA	Vowel Length	Example Word(s)
e, ea, ay	ɛ	short (s)	ever, head, **says**	er	ɚ	long	perfect, player
ey, a, ei	e	long (l)	ate, they, vein	ear, ur, ir	ɝ	short	earth, church, her, bird
i, ee, e	ɪ	short	if, been, English	ire	air	long	fire, squire, choir
e, ee, ie, ea	ɨ	long	eve, beef, chief, pea	our, or, au	ɔr	short	pour, oral, aura
u, oo, o	ʊ	short	pull, foot, woman	ar, ear	ɑr	long	car, heart
u, oo	u	long	rude, food	arr,	ær	long	arrow
u	ju	long	use, tube, fuse	ier, ear, eer	ɨr	short	pier, hear, peer
a, o,	ə	short (schwa)	about, award, oblige	err, er	ɛr	short	berry, merit
a, ou, u	ʌ	short	up, was, touch, but	air, are, ear	er	long	hair, bare, tear
a, o,	a	short	calm, job	oor, our	ur	long	poor, your
a, ai	æ	short	glad, plaid, have	ure	jur	long	cure, mural
o, a	ɑ	long	object, box, yacht	**Diphthongs**			
o, oa, ow, oe	o	long	coke, go, oath, low, toe	ai, i	ai	short	dime
aw, au, a, o	ɔ	short	saw, caught, all, off	oy	ɔɨ	short	boy
				ou	aʊ	short	out

Table 4–2. Consonant Legend (Spelling Variations)

Speech Sound	IPA	Example Word(s)	Speech Sound	IPA	Example Word(s)
p, pp, pe	p	**p**act, su**pp**er, ho**pe**	sh, ch, su, ti, ci	ʃ	**sh**e, **ch**ef, **s**ugar, a**c**tion, fa**ci**al
b, bb	b	**b**ad, ri**bb**on	si, s, g, z	ʒ	A**si**a, clo**s**ure, re**g**ime, sei**z**ure
k, c, ch, cc, ck, qu	k	**k**ey, **c**ab, a**ch**e, stu**cc**o, ba**ck**, anti**qu**e	m, mn, lm, mb	m	**m**ad, hy**mn**, pa**lm**, co**mb**
g, gg, gue	g	**g**o, e**gg**, ro**gue**	n, gn, kn, pn, ne	n	**n**ib, **gn**aw, **kn**it, **pn**eumonia, fi**ne**
th	θ	**th**ank, au**th**or	ng, ngue	ŋ	a**ng**er, sa**ng**, to**ngue**
th(dh), the	ð	**th**ose, **th**em, ba**the**	h, wh, j	h	**h**en, **wh**o, **B**aja
t, ght, th, te, ed	t	**t**ap, tau**ght**, **Th**eresa, vo**te**, pass**ed**	l, ll	l	**l**ad, ba**ll**
d, dd, ed, de	d	**d**am, a**dd**ing, stay**ed**, co**de**	f, ff, gh, ph	f	**f**an, cli**ff**, cou**gh**, **ph**one
s, c, ps, sc, sy	s	**s**it, **c**ell, **ps**alms, **sc**ene, **sy**mbol,	r, rr, rh	r	**r**ain, pu**rr**, co**rr**ect, **rh**yme
z, cz, zz, s, ss	z	**z**oo, **cz**ar, bu**zz**, lo**s**er, sci**ss**ors	v, f	v	**v**eal, o**f**
ch, tu	tʃ	**ch**ant, frac**tu**re	w, o, u	w	**w**ag, **o**nce, g**u**ava
g, j, ge, dge, gg	dʒ	**g**el, **j**elly, a**ge**, e**dge**, su**gg**est	y, eu, u, ll	j	**y**ak, **Eu**clid, **u**nite, torti**ll**a

Table 4–3. Vowel Sounds and Their IPA Symbols

e	e	i	i	u	u	u	o	o	a	a	a	u	a	ai	oy	ou
ɛ	e	ɪ	ɨ	ʊ	u	ju	o	ɔ	a	ɑ	æ	ʌ	ə	aɪ	ɔɨ	aʊ

Table 4–4. "r-Colored" Vowel Sounds and Their IPA Symbols

player	bird	choir	car	arrow	pour	hear	hair	berry	poor	cure
er	ur	ire	ar	are	or	ir	are	er	oor	yur
ɚ	ɝ	aɪr	ɑr	ær	ɔr	ɨr	er	ɛr	ur	jur

Table 4–5. Consonant Sounds and Their IPA Symbols

p	b	k	g	th	dh	t	d	s	z	ch	dz	sh	zh	m	n	ng	h	l	f	r	v	w	ya
p	b	k	g	θ	ð	t	d	s	z	tʃ	dʒ	ʃ	ʒ	m	n	ŋ	h	l	f	r	v	w	j

Demonstration of Phonetic Transcription

When the word is spelled phonetically using the IPA characters, you will be able to pronounce any word accurately and with ease. Without this information, you risk being misled either by an inadequately trained ear or by the "normal" spelling.

For example, compare the English spelling with the phonetic spelling or transcription for the word "suite." As a non-native speaker you probably would pronounce it the way it is spelled, saying "soot" with a long oo vowel sound and omitting the e sound altogether. However, if the word is represented using IPA symbols, the correct pronunciation is evident:

English spelling   **suite**

Phonetic transcription   **swɨt**

Ideally, for second language learners, the correct pronunciation of a word should be learned at the same time as when the word is incorporated into active vocabulary. So when you are learning the words "write," "rite," and "right," for example, should you pronounce them the way they are spelled? First, try saying them according to their spelling; notice any differences in pronunciation.

Now try using phonetic transcription. Phonetic transcription shows that all three words—"write," "rite," and "right"—are spoken the *exact* same way. The same three IPA symbols—**r** for the beginning r sound,

ai for the middle vowel sound (long i), and **t** for the ending t sound—are used:

write   **rait**

rite   **rait**

right   **rait**

Such words with the same pronunciation but different spellings are called *homophones.*

As another example, compare the pronunciations of ch in the words "chair" and "chemical." From Table 4–2, we see that ch in "chair" is the tʃ (IPA) sound and ch in "chemical" is the k (IPA) sound. Phonetically the words would be spelled as follows:

chair   **tʃer**

chemical   **kemɪkəl**

However, for a second language learner, the error in pronunciation could be **kər** or **tʃemikəl** because of confusion about whether to pronounce ch as **tʃ** or **k**. Essentially the only way to determine the difference in such instances is with practice.

Key Points in Transcription and Practice

Important points to remember about phonetic transcription are the following:

1. Phonetic transcription is based on use of the IPA, which consists of symbols for each speech sound that differ from the "normal" alphabet script (ABCs).

2. It is a process requiring familiarity with all of the different symbols, just as with the alphabet for any language.

3. Start by familiarizing yourself with each of the sounds in isolation.

4. Proceed to training your ears to auditory discrimination of each of the sounds using the symbols.

5. Concentrate on learning the vowel symbols and sounds first, because this is crucial to arrive at the "right" pronunciation of every word.

6. Learn a few consonant symbols and combine them with the vowel symbols to make familiar words.

7. Try to identify the speech sound you have learned within other words and write down its symbol.

8. The symbols must be memorized.

Review the examples in Table 4–6 carefully. Observe the spelling variations, scrutinize the IPA transcription, and, finally, pronounce each word *aloud*.

Table 4–6. Pronunciation Examples

English Spelling	IPA/Pronunciation
tight	taɪt
seat	sɨt
beverage	bɛʊrədʒ
acorn	ekorn
accent	æksɛnt
speaking	spɨkiŋ
railroad	reəlrod
Newark	njʊʌrk
retrospect	rɛtrospɛkt
New York	njʊ jɔrk
punctuality	pʌntʃʊælɪ<u>d</u>i (<u>t</u>)
acquittal	ʌkwɪtəl
newscast	nju<u>z</u>kæst (<u>s</u>)
equipment	ɛkwɪpmɛnt
Mississippi	mɪsəsɪpɪ
larynx	lærɪŋks
Connecticut	kʌnɛtɪkʌt
psychology	saɪkalədʒɨ
general	dʒɛnɚəl

Summary

Phonetic transcription at first is a painstaking process that takes you from symbols to pronunciation. It takes time to get acquainted with the different symbols, just as you learn the alphabet for any language, and then to put it into practice. Training your ears to critically distinguish between the sounds represented by the symbols is a challenge. It is worth repeating here that there are no shortcuts to learning the symbols—memorization of the symbols is a must. Again, patience and persistent practice constitute the key to success.

By now you probably have a good grasp of the symbol-sound concept of pronunciation: use of one symbol for each sound you hear or detect. However, other peculiarities of pronunciation often are noted in "running" or conversational speech. Such variations, which may arise without warning during fast conversational speech and influence the contextual cues or speech-sound assimilation, are discussed in detail in later chapters.

Begin your phonetic transcription practice using the worksheet that follows. Completing these drills will improve your competence in this skill so that you will be able to transcribe any word in an instant. Gradually add to your list of practice words. With mastery of phonetic transcription, any language becomes easy to learn.

Keep the tables of vowel and consonant legends handy as you practice the process of phonetic transcription.

WORKSHEET 4

Phonetic Transcription Practice

Instructions:

1. Keep the Vowel and Consonant Legends handy before you begin the practice of Phonetic transcription.

2. Listen to each of the words clearly. You have to use one symbol for each sound you hear or detect.

3. List the symbols you identified in the IPA transcription column.

4. Rewrite the IPA symbols together as a complete word in the third column provided.

5. Read the word aloud and monitor your pronunciation.

6. The exercises are organized under six headings; Mono/Disyllabic words, Multisyllabic words, Homophones, Homonyms, Phunnies in English pronunciation and your list of words for practice.

Mono and Disyllabic words

English Spelling	IPA Transcription	Pronunciation
alley		
ally		
mobile		
juvenile		
agile		
senile		

English Spelling	IPA Transcription	Pronunciation
white		
wait		
wet		
wheat		
eyebrow		
dial		
lawyer		
science		
signs		
however		
empower		
waver		
percent		
Xerox		
policeman		
enough		
stove		
refrigerator		

English Spelling	IPA Transcription	Pronunciation
pizza		
pizzazz		
digital		
diagnostic		

More words for Phonetic Transcription Practice

English Spelling	IPA Transcription	Pronunciation
quite		
quiet		
quit		
predict		
indict		
write		
written		
measure		
pressure		
tension		
clinician		

English Spelling	IPA Transcription	Pronunciation
shrubbery		
shredder		
expect		
aspect		
accept		
except		
beginner		
again		
train		
lever		
liver		
savior		
savor		
Sioux City		
Illinois		

Multisyllable Practice Words

English Spelling	IPA Transcription	Pronunciation
cemetery		
pentagon		
develop		
adhesive		
equipment		
Sioux City		
testimony		
subliminal		
reciprocal		
ability		
intelligibility		
responsibility		
practical		
spherical		
municipal		
decal		
delicatessen		
detour		

English Spelling	IPA Transcription	Pronunciation
competent		
component		
composite		
unbiased		
unreliable		
unavoidable		
silhouettes		
old-timers		
boyish		
irresistible		
irrefutable		
innumerable		

Homophones

These are words that sound alike but have different spellings. Example: write, rite, right.

English Spelling	IPA Transcription	Pronunciation
break		
brake		
pleural		
plural		

English Spelling	IPA Transcription	Pronunciation
site		
cite		
sight		
might		
mite		
bear		
bare		
bridle		
bridal		
vale		
veil		
flair		
flare		
pair		
pear		
see		
sea		

English Spelling	IPA Transcription	Pronunciation
racket		
racquet		
haul		
hall		

Homonyms

These are words that are spelled the same but sound different in different contexts.

English Spelling	IPA Transcription	Pronunciation
tear		
tear		
bow		
bow		
object		
object		
lead		
lead		
read		
read		

English Spelling	IPA Transcription	Pronunciation
wind		
wind		
wound		
wound		
minute		
minute		
resume		
resume		
putting		
putting		
bass		
bass		
live		
live		

Phunnies in English Pronunciation

English Spelling	IPA Transcription	Pronunciation
kind		
kindle		
debut		
often		
knack		
gnat		
talk		
film		
calm		
compass		
compassion		
photo		
photograph		
photography		
photogenic		
image		
imagine		
imagery		

English Spelling	IPA Transcription	Pronunciation
psychology		
psychological		
psychiatry		
allege		
allegation		
origin		
originate		
original		
nation		
national		
wild		
wilderness		

Your practice Words

English Spelling	IPA Transcription	Pronunciation

5

Speech Sounds: Vowels

Vowels represent an extremely important area of English phonology (speech sound production) because they are responsible for the greatest differences between the various spoken English dialects—that is, accents. It is worth emphasizing that it's the *vowel* within a word that holds the most information for the listener to help recognize and identify the word. Accordingly, it is very important to learn *how* the vowel sounds are made. In your accent management program, this knowledge will help you recognize the correct pronunciation of any word.

How are vowel sounds made? Let's try a quick exercise. First, take a seat in front of a mirror. Say a, e, i, o, u as you normally would. Now prolong each vowel for a few seconds, to exaggerate the sound production. Watch how your oral cavity changes shape. Try to *feel* the changes in your tongue position for each of the vowels, and notice that the tongue never actually obstructs the air flow. Use a mirror to follow the changes in shape as you move from vocalizing one vowel to another.

As you can see, the different vowel sounds are determined by changes in position of the lips, tongue, and palate. These changes can be very slight and difficult to detect. You have to train your hearing to help you identify and detect subtle differences between the vowel sounds. By contrast, during the production of consonant sounds, the lips, teeth, and other articulators are used to create various degrees and types of air flow obstruction in the vocal tract; the associated positional changes are readily seen.

What makes the vowels so important? For one thing, *vowel length* may be a decisive factor in vowel identification. In certain words, the length of the vowel—short or long—carries the stress information (discussed in later chapters) that is vital to the meaning. This allows the listener to discriminate between similar-sounding words, which in turn will enhance the clarity of the message. And with improved clarity, your message is understood, without your having to repeat yourself. Most importantly, whether your accent is erased or not, clarity is the ultimate goal in any conversation.

For example, compare the words "foot" and "food." In both words, the vowel o is doubled, to make a separate, unique sound, oo. But just as with the five original vowels (a, e, i, o, and u), the vowel combination oo also can be either short or long. In "foot," the vowel sound oo is *short* and its IPA phonetic symbol is ʊ; in "food," the vowel sound oo is *long*, with the IPA symbol u (refer to the Vowel Legend). Phonetic transcription gives /fʊt/ for "foot," with the short vowel sound, and /fud/ for "food," with a long vowel sound.

Let's say you interchanged the long and the short vowel sounds. Then /fʊt/ becomes /fut/—an incorrect pronunciation for "foot." If this interchange of the short and the long vowels between words occurs because of the influence of your native language, your pronunciation will deviate from the norms of Standard English. Then your speech will be heard as *accented English*.

Hence, an understanding of the nature of vowel sounds, not just the original five but all of the fourteen types, is essential for all learners of English as a second language (ESL). And learning the IPA script is essential to all second language learners all over the globe.

Vowel Portrait and Descriptions

Now let's go a little deeper into the world of vowels. To understand how vowel sounds are made, picture your mouth as a hollow tube whose walls are expandable, changing dimension for each vowel sound. Add in the movements of the tongue, lips, and jaw and changes in the degree of tension in the walls of this hollow tube—the oral cavity. The resulting differences in quality of sound are what enable you to distinguish one vowel from another.

The movements of the walls of the oral cavity and the articulators are not clearly visible, so the vowels have to be mastered through the process of auditory discrimination—differentiating between sounds by means of careful listening (the subject of Chapter 8)—and in context within a

conversation. Hence, vowels are far more difficult to transcribe phonetically than consonants.

The ability of the articulators to make subtle changes in the shape of the oral cavity is the basis for vowel production. Air escapes unobstructed through the mouth in the production of a vowel sound. Because there are no obvious obstructions, like those that characterize the production of consonants (such as in pressing lips together for /p/), it is difficult to categorize vowel sounds.

Hence, linguistic researchers have come up with creative ways to classify the vowels. Vowel classification is based on the following categories:

- where the tongue movements occur, i.e. raising of the tongue (front, center, back), raising toward the roof of the mouth, palate (high, mid, low), and the tension of the tongue (tense or lax)

- the length of time the vowel sound is held within words (long or short)

- the kind of opening made at the lips (retracted, rounded, or neutral)

The accompanying box lists the vowel sounds arranged according to the classification guidelines. Don't panic when you see the range of information presented; it will take some time to memorize the sounds and use them within your own speech.

As you begin to commit this information to memory, you will develop the ability to detect the subtle differences by training your sense of hearing. Perhaps you'll hear yourself speak and think: "That doesn't sound right!" Then you can refer to the vowel list to transcribe your speech. So this list is another tool you can use to measure your progress with foreign accent management.

Categories of Vowel Descriptions (includes "r-colored" vowels)

- The part of the tongue that is raised—front, center, or back

  Front vowels: i, ɪ, e, ɛ, æ

  Center vowels: ʌ, a, ir, er, or, ɝ, ar, air, ɚ

  Back vowels: u, ʊ, o, ɔ

- The degree to which the tongue rises in the direction of the palate (roof of the mouth)

  High: i, ɪ, u

  Mid: e, ɛ, ʌ, ɝ, ir, er, or, air, ʊ, o, ɚ

  Low: æ, a, ɔ

- The amount of tension in the tongue (affects vowel clarity)

  Tense: i, u, e, o, ɝ, ir, or, ar, air, er

  Lax: ɪ, ʊ, ɛ, ʌ, a, æ, ɚ, ɔ

- The length of time the vowel sound is held within words

  Long: i, u, e, o, ɝ, ir, or, ar, air, er

  Short: ɪ, ʊ, ɛ, ʌ, a, æ, ɚ, ɔ

- The kind of opening made at the lips—various degrees of lip rounding and spreading (may be the only visual clue to assist in vowel identification)

  Retracted lips: i, ɪ, e, ɛ, æ

  Rounded lips: u, ʊ, o, ɔ

  Neutral lips: ʌ, a, ɚ

Diphthongs

Recall that certain vowels repeated twice make a separate, unique vowel sound (a double o, for example, makes oo, with *two* possible sounds!). In other vowel sounds, two *different* vowels combine. These sounds are called *diphthongs*.

A diphthong is a combination of two vowels in which the spoken sound glides from one vowel sound to another. There is a smooth changeover as the articulators (lips, tongue, and so on) adjust their tension so that the sound of one vowel imperceptibly merges with the sound of a second vowel. Try pronouncing the following examples:

/ɔɪ/ as in "**boy**": [bɔɪ]

/aʊ/ as in "**mouth**": [maʊth]

/aɪ/ as in "**fly**": [flaɪ]

Vowels, Spelling, and Pronunciation

Each vowel sound has a standard spelling pattern that is based on its frequency of use in the English language (the spelling that is used more often than any other acceptable version is considered the official, standard spelling). However, there are various ways in which vowel sounds are represented by the letters of the alphabet.

For example, say the words "hear" and "bear." They are both spelled with **ea** as the vowel sound. Yet the **ea** in "hear" is the /i/ sound (long e), whereas the **ea** in "bear" is the /e/ sound (long a). Similarly, each vowel sound has other spelling variations (see Table 4–1); these are addressed in practice exercises later in this chapter.

Phonetic versus Alphabetic Vowel Sounds

Table 5–1 lists all of the vowels in the International Phonetic Alphabet, along with the "normal" alphabet symbols. Vowel spelling variations are listed in Chapter Four (Table 4–1). There are no shortcuts to learning the symbols—they must be *memorized*.

Table 5–1. Vowels in Alphabetic and IPA Symbols

Vowel Legend			
Speech Sound	**IPA**	**IPA in Words**	**English Spelling**
e	ɛ	bɛd	bed
a	e	bek	bake
i	ɪ	bɪt	bit
i	ɨ	bɨt	beat
u	ʊ	bʊk	book
u	u	but	boot
u	ju	bjutɪ	beauty
o	o	bow	bow
ou	ɔ	bɔght	bought
o	a	balm	balm
a	ɑ	bɑx	box
a	æ	bæd	bad
u	ʌ	bʌt	but
a	ə	əbout	about

The Cardinal Vowel System

There are many other ways of classifying vowel sounds. Several phonetic transcriptions to indicate various usages of vowels have been devised, based on different interpretations by language scientists. The Cardinal Vowel System was devised by a British phonetician, Daniel Jones (1881–1967). This system is widely used in the field of speech-language pathology. The Cardinal Vowel System is shown in Figure 5–1.

Summary

Now you have an idea of the importance of vowels within words. An important principle in accent management is that it is the *vowel* within a word that holds the most information for the listener to help identify the word. If vowels sounds are perfected, speech clarity is automatically enhanced.

Vowels act as vehicles to carry us toward the right pronunciation. So it is imperative to learn *how* the vowels sounds are made. Be-

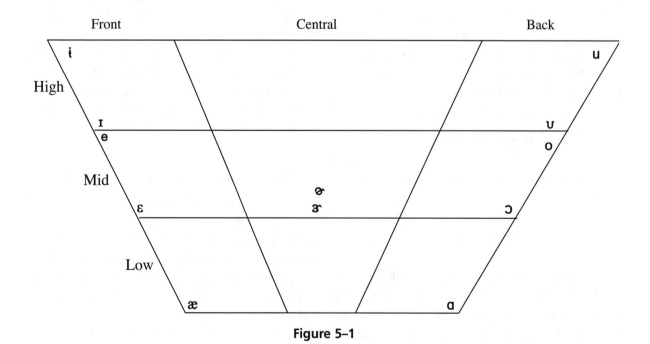

Figure 5–1

sides understanding the basic vowel descriptions of short-long, tense-lax, you need to pay attention to spelling variations because spelling directly affects pronunciation.

Learning phonetic symbols is another integral component of the process of accent management. Thorough familiarity with the phonetic symbols will make it easier to identify the correct vowel sound within each word, thereby assisting in the correct pronunciation and leading to appropriate accent management.

Here are some tips for practice:

1. Use the Vowel Legend (Table 4–1) to memorize the sounds and compare the differences between the sounds.

2. Read the listed words aloud.

3. Listen carefully to the vowel sound in each of the words.

4. Listen critically to how each vowel sound changes from one word to another.

5. Use a mirror for feedback to watch the movements of your articulators.

Now you are ready to tackle the practice exercises on vowels in the worksheets at the end of this chapter. Don't be alarmed at the number of worksheets. There's usually just one page for each sound, with exercises starting from words and progressing to sentences.

WORKSHEET 5

Speech Sounds: Vowels

Instructions:

1. Vowel sounds are divided into the following patterns of units for targeted practice.
   - /a/ and /o/ variations
   - Diphthongs
   - /j/ sound as in yellow
   - Paired Vowels (/u/ and /ʊ/, /i/and /ɪ/, /e/ and /ɛ/
   - Sentences for Long and Short vowels
   - Vowels—IPA transcription
   - r-colored vowels

2. Say each vowel sound individually to identify the manner of production. Paying attention to how and where (in the oral cavity) the individual vowel sounds are made assists you in identifying the "right" vowel sound within any word.

Vowel Legend

e	e	i	i	u	u	u	o	o	a	a	a	u	a	ai	oy	ou
ɛ	e	ɪ	ɨ	ʊ	u	ju	o	ɔ	a	ɑ	æ	ʌ	ə	aɪ	ɔɪ	aʊ

3. Pay close attention to the short (s) and long (l) vowel sounds.

4. Say the vowels for front to back and feel the placement within your mouth: /ɨ/, /a/, /o/, /ɔ/

5. Feel the contrast between "front" and "back" sounds as you repeat the following vowels: /ɨ/ and /u/, /e/ and /o/.

6. High/low vowel contrasts: /ɨ/ and /a/, /u/ and /o/

7. Repeat all the "front" vowels and feel how your articulation position moves from high to low.

8. Long and short vowels: /ɨ/ and /ɪ/, /u/ and /ʊ/, /e/ and /ɛ/

9. Feel the tongue tension change as you repeat the following vowels: /ɨ/ and /ɪ/, /u/ and /ʊ/, /e/ and /ɛ/.

10. Observe the lips retracting and rounding as you repeat the following vowels: /u/ and /ʊ/, /o/ and /e/, /a/ and /o/, /æ/ and /ɔ/.

11. Practice the steps two through ten multiple times until production of vowels feels comfortable. You can gradually progress to the practice of speech drills for each of the vowel sounds.

The following table lists the phonetic alphabet forms followed by examples. You may have to memorize a target word for each vowel sound to help with phonetic transcription.

ʌ	as in "sun" "but"	o	as in "coke"
æ	as in "thank"	ɔ	as in "all," "call"
a	as in "calm"	ai	as in "time"
ɑ	as in "box"	aʊ	as in "out"
ə	as in "about"	ɔi	as in "boy"

Speech drills include practice lists of simple/common words, multisyllable words, and sentences. Notes on any variations in spelling, with relevant lists, are included as well.

/ʌ/ and /o/

/ʌ/ as in "sun," "but"

Words with /ʌ/ Sound

bud	pun	hut	buck	bulb
thud	run	shut	struck	bulk
hug	up	cuff	mush	must
plug	pup	huff	flush	crust
fund	bump	duct	munch	lust
hunk	stump	cult	crunch	bulge

Multisyllable Words with /ʌ/

bucket	sculpture	buttoning	discussion	wonderfully
subject	rummaging	interrupting	smothering	discovery
luckiest	thundering	impulsive	beloved	conductor
suctioning	junction	adjustment	tongue	justice
suddenly	deduction	somewhere	government	shuttling
struggling	compulsion	eruption	recovering	puzzlement

/ʌ/ Spelling Variations

The /ʌ/ sound has the spelling variations **ou**, **a**, **au**, **oe**, and **oo**. Examples: **ou** as in "trouble," "cousin," "southern"; **a** as in "what"; **au** as in "because," "authority"; **oe** as in "does"; **oo** as in "flood." However, not all words with these letter combinations are pronounced with the /ʌ/ sound. Compare the words **rou**te and **trou**ble, **does** and **toe**, and **foo**d and **floo**d.

Practice Sentences with /ʌ/

Find the words with the /c/ sound within the following sentences.

1. The janitor was asked to shut the duct.
2. Did you donate to your favorite fund?
3. It is dangerous to make impulsive decisions.
4. Please don't interrupt the conductor during practice.
5. She was munching on the pizza crust.
6. Suddenly the discussion about sculptures ended.
7. The government made new rules about deductions.
8. She is recovering from surgery.
9. She bumped into her high school classmate at the mall.
10. What is the schedule for the shuttle service?

Your Sentences with /ʌ/

Make up your own sentences using /ʌ/ words from one of the preceding lists.

1. _____

2. _____

3. _____

4. _____

5. _____

/æ/ as in "bat," "thank"

Words with /æ/ Sound

scab	gal	cap	flat	tax
bad	pal	clap	sat	as
dad	shall	wrap	snack	has
glad	glass	ash	back	mass
add	grass	crash	bang	bath
craft	band	ranch	slang	wrath

Multisyllable Words with /æ/

cabbage	glamorous	passionate	exaggerate	satisfaction
fraction	management	managerial	maximum	examination
language	mannerisms	janitorial	reactive	graduation
standard	sampling	accidental	romantic	battered
tanbark	entangle	nationality	detachment	championship
balance	languish	fashionable	attachment	snapdragon

/æ/ Spelling Variations

The /æ/ sound has other spellings: **ai**, **au**, and **a** + one or more consonants + **e**. Examples: **ai** as in "plaid"; **au** as in "aunt," "laugh"; and **a** + consonant + **e** as in "have," "giraffe." However, not all words with these letter combinations are pronounced with a /æ/ sound. Compare the words r**ai**d and pl**ai**d, **au**thor and **au**nt, and c**afe** (café) and gir**affe**.

Practice Sentences with /æ/

Find the words with the /æ/ sound within the following sentences.

1. That gal has a white cap.
2. Please wrap the gift for Dad's birthday.
3. We are glad that you were not hurt in the crash.
4. Get your snack and a glass of milk.
5. The management took glamorous vacations.
6. His language and mannerisms were different from ours.
7. What is your nationality?

8. Her mother looked happy and proud on the day of her graduation.

9. He has just a fraction of his balance left in his account.

10. Practice detachment instead of attachment.

Your Sentences with /æ/

Make up your own sentences using /æ/ words from one of the preceding lists.

1. _____

2. _____

3. _____

4. _____

5. _____

/a/ as in "calm"

Words with /a/ Sound

aqua	macho	launch	yard	calmer
father	nacho	jaunt	watt	gazpacho
balm	pasta	wand	want	swab
mama	salsa	psalm	watch	farm
palm	part	staunch	what	dharma
papa	spa	yacht	squat	llama

Multisyllable Words with /a/

pajamas	swapping	watchman	quantity	facade
qualm	wristwatch	wandering	quality	mirage
drama	swallow	squabble	qualify	corsage
suave	garage	sabotage	massage	collage
palmistry	barrage	quadrant	pardon	watering
darling	embark	salary	marmalade	pharmacy

/a/ Spelling Variations

The /a/ sound has various spellings in addition to the usual **a**: **au** as in "aunt" (British English), "jaunt"; **a** after w, wh, sw, qu, and squ, in "watt," "what," "swap," "qualify," and "squad"; **a** + consonant + **e** as in "collage." However, not all words with these letter combinations are pronounced with the /a/ sound. Compare the words j**au**nt and **au**rora, qu**a**ke and qu**a**drangle, coll**a**ge and ch**a**fe.

Practice Sentences with /a/

Find the words with the /a/ sound within the following sentences.

1. Mama Rosa makes good homemade salsa.
2. She needed a wand to complete her costume.
3. He bought an expensive watch for her birthday.
4. He owns a luxurious yacht.
5. She is a staunch believer in vegetarianism.
6. The drama center was offering summer classes.
7. Why are you wandering along the corridors?
8. Which pharmacy do you use?
9. Take your squabbles to the garage.
10. Did you qualify for a car loan?

Your Sentences with /a/

Make up sentences using /a/ words from one of the preceding lists.

1. _____
2. _____
3. _____
4. _____
5. _____

/a/ as in "box"

Spread your lips when saying the /a/ sound within words.

Words with /a/ Sound

job	ox	notch	lodge	shop
object	boss	bond	mom	top
odd	bob	chop	not	Tom
nod	copy	font	pomp	topic
God	throb	fox	rot	robin
con	plot	got	pond	rotten

Multisyllable Words with /a/

honest	optical	spotted	dollar	positive
olive	onstage	follow	operate	option
colossal	responsible	body	phonic	compact
bombard	snobbish	bottle	economic	context
probably	compound	correspond	novel	topnotch
possible	involve	nonsense	popular	monstrous

/a/ Spelling Variations

The vowel sound /a/ does not have other spellings.

Practice Sentences with /a/

Find the words with the /a/ sound within the following sentences.

1. What are the objects inside this box?
2. Please chop some vegetables for a salad.
3. Have you been rock climbing?
4. Her eyes were bombarded with optical illusions in the lab.
5. You have to knock twice at his door.
6. Follow your body's cues during all exercise routines.
7. Are you responsible to present other options?

8. She operated her business on a tight budget.

9. The model had to sing a song onstage.

10. She spotted the lost correspondence under a pile on her desk.

Your Sentences with /ɑ/

Make up your own sentences using /ɑ/ words from one of the preceding lists.

1. _____

2. _____

3. _____

4. _____

5. _____

/ə/ as in "about"

Words with /ə/ Sound

abide	adopt	appease	fatigue	convict
accord	astute	galore	attest	conflict
accrue	alarm	ascribe	attire	consult
aboard	alert	aspire	afford	contest
attach	allege	cassette	adjust	object
address	amass	assort	avoid	command

Multisyllable Words with /ə/

appraisal	attendance	alignment	lapel	patrolman
avenged	appointment	annulment	lacrosse	possession
adjourned	caboose	contempt	legitimate	pollution
acquainted	approach	canoe	machinery	rapport
achiever	bazaar	offensive	maturity	submission
salute	severe	chagrin	velour	maternity

/ə/ Spelling Variations

The /ə/ sound has other spellings: **o** as in "occur," "complete," and **u** as in "subject," "suggest."

Practice Sentences with /ə/

Find the words with the /ə/ sound within the following sentences.

1. One has to abide by the rules of an institution or company.
2. Please attach a cover letter to your resume.
3. Be aboard the ship by 9 AM sharp.
4. Can everyone afford the "American Dream"?
5. His ear canal was occluded.
6. The patrolman commanded the cyclist to stop.
7. Are you acquainted with the Masons?
8. Your appointment was at 6 PM yesterday.
9. She looked at the lawyer in contempt.
10. His comment to the child was offensive.

Your Sentences with /ə/

Make up your own sentences using /ə/ words from one of the preceding lists.

1. _____

2. _____

3. _____

4. _____

5. _____

/o/ as in "go," "coke"

Words with /o/ Sound

old	owe	colt	tone	open
scold	bow	gross	close	soda
odor	flow	host	quote	focus
omit	grown	robe	prose	vocal
opaque	control	code	drove	hero
overt	poll	smoke	froze	auto

Multisyllable Words with /o/

folder	showplace	postage	notary	custodian
withhold	overthrow	foremost	location	approach
shareholder	swollen	lonely	robust	milestone
boastful	payroll	provoke	promotion	outspoken
donation	enrollment	explode	foreclose	opponent
photograph	wholesale	modem	monotone	portfolio

/o/ Spelling Variations

The /o/ sound has other spellings: **eau** as in "beau"; **oa** as in "oath," "load"; **ough** as in "dough"; **ou** as in "shoulder"; **ew** as in "sew"; **au** as in "taupe," "chauffeur."

Practice Sentences with /o/

Find the words with the /o/ sound within the following sentences.

1. How old is the host?
2. Take a stroll in the park after dinner.
3. Mr. Brown seems to have grown older in the past year.
4. Focus on your prose instead of poetry.
5. Has the payroll department been notified of the error?
6. Did you get that promotion?
7. They did not withhold enough taxes this year.
8. Her mom froze when she saw Sandy smoking.

9. What is her role in this play?

10. When does the enrollment begin?

Your Sentences with /o/

Make up your own sentences using /o/ words from one of the preceding lists.

1. _____

2. _____

3. _____

4. _____

5. _____

/ɔ/ as in "all," "call"

Words with /ɔ/ Sound

always	dogma	waltz	haughty	stalk
audit	fought	wallet	lofty	faucet
offer	gone	yawn	strong	prongs
off-shoot	gawky	squaw	glossy	broth
often	pauper	crawl	squash	straws
boss	wrong	stall	honk	gauze

Multisyllable Words with /ɔ/

augment	faultless	vaulted	haunting	exhaustion
awestruck	saucer	awkward	auctioneer	manslaughter
almanac	frosting	auditorium	drawstring	hallmark
altogether	cross-guard	assaulted	distraught	falsehood
smoggy	haunting	authenticated	saucepan	auspicious
softener	belongings	unlawful	long-range	offhand

/ɔ/ Spelling Variations

The /ɔ/ sound has several spelling variations: **au** as in "fault," **aw** as in "shawl," **oa** as in broad," **ou** as in "cough."

Practice Sentences with /ɔ/

Find the words with the /ɔ/ sound within the following sentences.

1. Do you always get audited?
2. Don't crawl under the bed.
3. She was awestruck by Hong Kong.
4. She had to honk to get the kid off the street.
5. There was flooding because of 10 inches of rainfall.
6. She felt awkward in her new dress.
7. Why are you stalling?
8. Make some tossed salad and pasta for dinner.
9. Where is the auditorium?
10. He was being sentenced for manslaughter.

Your Sentences with /ɔ/

Make up your own sentences using /ɔ/ words from one of the preceding lists.

1. _____
2. _____
3. _____
4. _____
5. _____

Diphthongs

/ɔɪ/ as in "boy"

Words with /ɔɪ/ Sound

boil	doily	hoist	goiter	join
jointly	coy	coin	lawyer	loyal
moist	noise	point	poise	ploy
void	toilet	toys	toil	spoil
loiter	coil	soil	joist	annoy
enjoy	oyster	alloy	convoy	foyer

Multisyllable Words with /ɔɪ/

ointment	boyfriend	joyride	moisture	noise-proof
boycott	choiceness	coyness	poisonous	royally
moisten	noiseless	pointed	soybean	voiceprint
toyshop	broiled	buoyant	oilcan	hoisted
flamboyant	employer	disloyal	annoyance	enjoyment
exploited	adjoining	disappointment	boisterous	tenderloin

/ɔɪ/ Spelling Variations

The /ɔɪ/ sound may be spelled either **oi** as in "boil" or **oy** as in "coy."

Practice Sentences with /ɔɪ/

Find the words with the /ɔɪ/ sound within the following sentences.

1. Do you have a joint bank account?
2. We have an appointment with the lawyer.
3. Draw a line through the check and mark it void.
4. Are you enjoying those oysters?
5. Her boyfriend needed an ointment for that rash.
6. She pointed out that the leaves were poisonous.
7. The employees decided to boycott the meeting.

8. Did you destroy all the work just to avoid publicity?

9. He was exploited by his employer.

10. This tree needs moist soil to grow.

Your Sentences with /ɔɪ/

Make up your own sentences using /ɔɪ/ words from one of the preceding lists.

1. _____

2. _____

3. _____

4. _____

5. _____

/a/ as in "time"

Words with /aɪ/ Sound

aisle	icon	child	diaper	height
either	bike	dial	file	hyper
ibis	buy	fiber	guide	jive
giant	lice	mine	mild	nylon
knife	night	pipe	python	rhyme
right	silent	silo	shine	tyke

Multisyllable Words with /aɪ/

cayenne	dilate	righteous	psychic	sign-off
sidekick	migraine	prescribe	oblige	confinement
pantomime	spitefully	paradise	patronize	compromise
subscriber	survival	privately	milestone	lightweight
vitamin	violent	typewriter	bronchitis	assignments
knee-high	guidance	delightful	highway	indictment

/ai/ Spelling Variations

The /ai/ sound may be spelled as shown in the lists: **ai**, **ia**, **ei**, or **igh**, in addition to plain letter **i**. /ai/ also has spelling variations in final positions: **ie** as in "pie," **i** as in "hi," **y** as in "cry," and **i** followed by a consonant + **e** as in "tribe" "trite." Other variants are **ay** as in "cayenne" and **uy** as in "buy," "guy."

Practice Sentences with /aɪ/

Find the words with the /aɪ/ sound within the following sentences.

1. Did the tax collector take a bribe?
2. How many miles was your bike ride?
3. In spite of the notice, he was late.
4. This child is hyperactive at night.
5. He stayed silent, indicating compromise.
6. Are you working overtime on the pantomime project?
7. She took typewriting classes when she was nine.
8. Did the butterfly migrate from China?
9. The New York Public Library is a paradise for bookworms.
10. Can you modify your last assignment?

Your Sentences with /aɪ/

Make up your own sentences using /aɪ/ words from one of the preceding lists.

1. _____
2. _____
3. _____
4. _____
5. _____

/aʊ/ as in "out"

Words with /aʊ/ Sound

ouch	owlet	chowder	down	gout
howl	couch	lounge	coward	mouse
mouth	powder	route	rowdy	south
shout	towel	tower	thousand	vow
thou	drought	devout	how	owl
count	mount	flour	scowl	bout

Multisyllable Words/Phrases with /aʊ/

scoundrel	hourglass	boundary	warehouse	housewife
mountaineer	pronounce	surrounding	greyhound	discounted
voucher	trousers	birdhouse	throughout	allowance
pow-wow	empowering	endowment	powerful	somehow
eyebrow	horsepower	downtown	traumatic	sauerkraut
outrageous	encountering	counselors	"holy cow"	anyhow

/aʊ/ Spelling Variations

As shown in the word lists, the /aʊ/ sound is spelled **ou** as in "out" or **ow** as in "bow-wow." Some words spelled with **au** may also be pronounced with the /aʊ/ sound, such as "trauma."

Practice Sentences with /aʊ/

Find the words with the /aʊ/ sound within the following sentences.

1. He was on the couch with a scowl on his face.
2. His spouse is waiting in the lounge.
3. Count the steps all the way to the top of the tower.
4. Do you take Route 23 south to the park?
5. His office is in downtown Philadelphia.
6. She has to pick up her trousers from the cleaners.
7. It is a traumatic experience to lose your family in an accident.

8. Surrounding the house is a beautiful garden.

9. How do you pronounce this word?

10. She took the Greyhound to travel throughout the country.

Your Sentences with /aʊ/

Make up your own sentences using /aʊ/ words from one of the preceding lists.

1. _____

2. _____

3. _____

4. _____

5. _____

/j/ as in "yellow"

This is the /ya/ sound.

1. Start by placing the articulators in the relaxed "i" position.

2. The tongue tip is raised toward the palate (roof of the mouth) but does not touch it.

3. Give a slight forward movement to the jaw.

4. Terminate with /a/ sound.

5. Stress the "pose" till it feels comfortable.

6. Practice /j/ in individual words in initial and medial positions.

7. Graduate to sentences when you are ready.

Words/Phrases with /j/ in Initial, Medial, and Final Positions

In this and other similar word lists, supply IPA symbols for phonetic transcription of each term. An example has been done for you.

Initial	IPA	Medial	IPA	Final	IPA
yolk	jok	buoyant		papaya	
yield		New York City		Kenya	
yours		teriyaki		Maya	
young		Himalayas		Tanya	
youth		Scotland Yard			

Multisyllable Words/Initial and Medial Positions with /j/

Initial	IPA	Medial	IPA
yacht club		New York	
year-round		New Year's Eve	
yardstick		courtyard	
yearlong		loyalty	
Yorkshire		royalty	

/j/ Exceptions

English Spelling	IPA	English Spelling	IPA
articulate		ukulele	
Australia		eulogy	
savior		failure	
annual		unanimous	
figure		Ukraine	

/j/ Blend in the First Syllable

English Spelling	IPA	English Spelling	IPA	English Spelling	IPA
beauty		fjord		pure	
bugle		funeral		pupil	
curious		feud		view	
cucumber		Hugh		humane	
cupid		fume		new	

/j/ Blend in the Second Syllable

English Spelling	IPA	English Spelling	IPA	English Spelling	IPA
compute		manual		vacuum	
immune		menu		volume	
amuse		rescue		genuine	
debut		review		tribute	
commute		secure		acupuncture	

/j/ Blend in the Third Syllable

English Spelling	IPA	English Spelling	IPA	English Spelling	IPA
attribute		interview		minuscule	
barbecue		intramural		manipulative	
continue		manicure		therapeutic	
contribution		evacuation		vestibule	
evaluate		pedicure		executive	

Your List of /j/ Words

Initial	IPA	Medial	IPA	Final	IPA

Practice Sentences with /j/

1. The neighborhood yard sale is held annually.
2. Tom Yardley lives in New York City.
3. Have you visited Kenya?
4. Their contribution to the community is commendable.
5. Ewing travels to Uruguay on business.
6. Her Royal Highness Queen Maya wanted to eat papaya.
7. Eunice lives on Euclid Avenue.
8. Virginia is a young graduate from Yale.
9. The mayor of Yonkers was supportive of the governor's decision.
10. The ballplayer hired a lawyer to defend him.
11. It is our duty to preserve the environment for future generations.
12. Muriel went to a museum in Munich.
13. That young Malayan architect belongs to the Royal Family.
14. The chicken teriyaki was delicious.
15. Johannes delivered an excellent eulogy.
16. An anonymous executive made a generous contribution.
17. She had an appointment for a manicure and a pedicure.
18. Please continue your acupuncture treatment.
19. He was immune to the stress of long commuting.
20. Her speech was very articulate.

Short and Long Vowel Sounds: /ʊ/ and /u/, /ɪ/ and /ɨ/, /ɛ/ and /e/

/ʊ/ and /u/ as in "foot" and "food"

Words with /ʊ/ and /u/ Sounds

/ʊ/	/u/	/ʊ/	/u/	/ʊ/	/u/	/ʊ/	/u/
good	goose	hoof	hoop	pulled	pooled	wood	wooed
pull	pool	cook	cool	bull	boo	could	cooed
look	Luke	book	boot	full	fool	should	shooed
roof	root	push	poop	nook	nude	shook	shoot
full	food	took	tool	took	toot	crook	crude

Multisyllable Words with /ʊ/ and /u/

bullet	booster	cushion	foolproof	superb	movement
bully	bootie	crooked	goof-off	sugar	toothpaste
brook	booming	football	jewel	footstep	movie
bulldozer	boost	footprint	coolant	understood	newborn
booklet	dew	pudding	cuckoo	wooden	roommate

Practice Sentences with /ʊ/ and /u/

1. This tea is good for you.
2. That box is full.
3. There is a goose in the yard.
4. I cannot fool you!
5. Give the rope a pull.
6. I watched a football game today.
7. Do you have a pool?
8. Did he feel foolish at the meeting?
9. He is working on the roof.
10. Are you going to Sue's cookout?

/ɪ/ and /i/ as in "bit" and "beet"

Words with /ɪ/ and /i/ Sounds

/ɪ/	/i/	/ɪ/	/i/	/ɪ/	/i/	/ɪ/	/i/
sit	seat	quick	queen	knit	neat	pick	peek
if	eve	quill	sheer	sip	seep	rip	reap
ill	eel	rim	ream	ship	sheep	till	teal
mill	meal	spit	speak	lick	leek	sill	seal
nil	kneel	Sid	seed	tick	meek	slick	sleek

Multisyllable Words with /ɪ/ and /i/

beyond	beachwear	beeping	kneecap	peanut	release
eject	become	excited	business	meeting	rewind
equipment	beaten	exchange	election	written	meantime
evening	needle	beaming	neatness	ridden	prison
estate	enough	neon	silver	peaceful	weeping

Practice Sentences with /ɪ/ and /i/

1. Is that seat taken?
2. Will you go to the park with me?
3. Why don't you sit down?
4. "Wheel of Fortune" is on at seven-thirty.
5. Please take this pill once a day.
6. The faucet sprung a leak.
7. Can you peel the banana, please?
8. Go ahead and lick your ice cream cone.
9. Does he work at the mill?
10. The tins were in the other room.

/ɛ/ and /e/ as in "bet" and "baby"

Words with /ɛ/ and /e/ Sounds

/ɛ/	/e/	/ɛ/	/e/	/ɛ/	/e/	/ɛ/	/e/
egg	acorn	bed	Kate	berry	made	ledge	tail
elephant	pace	when	bait	leapt	paper	chef	day
else	raise	any	able	swept	nation	etch	navy
send	paint	belt	eight	baste	rate	twelve	cape
zest	glaze	clever	tame	bacon	pale	texture	lady

Multisyllable Words with /ɛ/ and /e/

sketching	maybe	seminar	today	emphasize	prostate
death	mainly	pessimist	orate	empathy	payment
threat	agency	restaurant	prostrate	development	basic
breakfast	alias	sledge	agent	emboli	daily
everlasting	area	metropolis	capable	petrified	grateful

Practice Sentences with /ɛ/ and /e/

1. Maybe Kate is looking for a job at the agency today.
2. What did the professor say about your grade?
3. Did you find your bracelet?
4. Please show some empathy toward Drake.
5. Drake meant what he said.
6. She is an angel to care for her grandmother.
7. Angel was upset about her dog's death.
8. Is Kate capable of networking in the metropolis?
9. This texture feels like rayon.
10. What was he arrested for in El Paso?

Practice Sentences with Long and Short Vowels

In the following sentences, underline the indicated vowel sounds and identify them as short (s) or long (l). The first one in each set has been done as an example.

/ɪ/ and /i/

1. The *seating is* for twent*y*. (l) (s) (s)
2. What if it happens?
3. That is breach of contract.
4. Bring me the blue folder labeled Mr. Reed.
5. Meet me at three to discuss the project.

/ʊ/ and /u/

1. It was *too good to* be *true*. (l) (s) (s) (l)
2. He looked at the full moon with childish excitement.
3. I heard footsteps upstairs.
4. Do you need coolant for your car?
5. Her hands shook when she held the packet.

/ɛ/ and /e/

1. *Abe went* apple picking *yester*day. (l) (s) (s) (l)
2. Kate thought that it was a sane thing to do.
3. Save these pictures for Ed.
4. Leah is leaning toward a summer wedding.
5. She stood at the doorway waving goodbye.

Vowel Sounds: IPA Transcription

Add IPA phonetic symbols for each of the vowel sounds within the following words or phrases. The first one has been done for you.

bullet	beeping	cushion	embarrass	superb	movement
/ʊ/, /ɛ/					
bully	excited	crook	sending	sugar	toothpaste
brook	exchange	football	measurement	shook	movie
bulldozer	beaming	footprint	treasure	understood	newborn
bookcase	because	footstep	or else	woman	newscast
rating	dew	meantime	stiff	today's	booklet
slate	duke	image	steep	orator	brushfire
slaying	dewdrop	neither	written	prostrate	cookbook
May Day	doodling	neon	ridden	agents	cooker
braying	foolish	listen	leaving	professor	cookout
roommate	booster	kneecap	cuckoo	release	seminars

Vowel Sounds: Overview

Identify *each* of the vowel sounds within the following sentences.

1. It was too good to be true.
2. He looked at the portrait in amazement.
3. I heard footsteps upstairs.
4. Do you need coolant for your car?
5. Did you watch figure skating last night?

"r - colored" Vowel Sounds

/er/, /or/ = /ɚ/

1. Raise the central part of the tongue halfway toward the roof of the mouth (palate).

2. The tongue tip should be raised to rest just behind the front teeth (alveolar ridge).

3. The lips are relaxed, not rounded, and open slightly.

4. Stress your "pose" to get it right and repeat multiple times till it feels comfortable.

5. Practice the sound in words using IPA transcription.

6. Make up sentences using the same words for more practice.

Words with /ɚ/

Medial	IPA	Final	IPA
lowering		drier	
powerboat		buyer	
showering		layer	
diapering		shower	

Your List of /ɚ/ Words

Medial	IPA	Final	IPA

Words with /ier/ = /iɚ/

Final	IPA
barrier	
courier	
meteor	
anterior	

Your List of /iɚ/ Words

Final	IPA

Words with /bɚ/

Medial	IPA	Final	IPA
hamburger		barber	
liberal		labor	
harboring		sober	
neighborhood		October	

Your List of /bɚ/ Words

Medial	IPA	Final	IPA

Words with /mber/ = /mbɚ/

Medial	IPA	Final	IPA
cumbersome		chamber	
		September	
		timber	
		slumber	

Your List of /mbɚ/ Words

Medial	IPA	Final	IPA

Words with /cher/ = /tʃɚ/

Medial	IPA	Final	IPA
archery		butcher	
cultural		capture	
naturalistic		launcher	
adventurous		preacher	

Your List of /tʃɚ/ Words

Medial	IPA	Final	IPA

Words with /der/ = /dɚ/

Medial	IPA	Final	IPA
orderly		cider	
thunderclap		ladder	
underneath		calendar	
powdering		ambassador	

Your List of /dɚ/ Words

Medial	IPA	Final	IPA

Words with /fer/ = /fɚ/

Medial	IPA	Final	IPA
different		camphor	
inference		golfer	
suffering		roofer	
conferring		wafer	

Your List of /fɚ/ Words

Medial	IPA	Final	IPA

Words with /ger/ = /gɚ/

Medial	IPA	Final	IPA
staggering		beggar	
rigorous		cougar	
vigorous		dagger	
eagerness		cheeseburger	

Your List of /gɚ/ Words

Medial	IPA	Final	IPA

Words with /ler/ = /lɚ/

Medial	IPA	Final	IPA
allergic		caller	
colorful		peddler	
gallery		angular	
salary		tricolor	

Your List of /lɚ/ Words

Medial	IPA	Final	IPA

Words with /ker/ = /kɚ/

Medial	IPA	Final	IPA
bakery		acre	
anchored		locker	
conquering		saltshaker	
licorice		soccer	

Your List of /kɚ/ Words

Medial	IPA	Final	IPA

Words with /mer/ = /mɚ/

Medial	IPA	Final	IPA
armory		farmer	
emerald		primer	
humerus		shimmer	
limerick		consumer	

Your List of /mɚ/ Words

Medial	IPA	Final	IPA

Words with /ner/ = /nɚ/

Medial	IPA	Final	IPA
energized		cleaner	
generosity		beginner	
runner-up		minor	
scenery		sooner	

Your List of /nɚ/ Words

Medial	IPA	Final	IPA

Words with /per/ = /pɚ/

Medial	IPA	Final	IPA
aspirin		gripper	
drapery		pepper	
property		stupor	
experiment		trooper	

Your List of /pɚ/ Words

Medial	IPA	Final	IPA

Words with /rɚ/

Final	IPA
error	
juror	
admirer	
conjurer	

Your List of /rɚ/ Words

Final	IPA

Words with /sher/ = /ʃɚ/

Medial	IPA	Final	IPA
fisherman		kosher	
pressurizing		masher	
washer/dryer		washer	
Glacier Bay		publisher	

Your List of /ʃɚ/ Words

Medial	IPA	Final	IPA

Words with /ster/ = /stɚ/

Medial	IPA	Final	IPA
asterisk		blister	
prehistoric		fluster	
masterful		pastor	
northeasterly		canister	

Your List of /stɚ/ Words

Medial	IPA	Final	IPA

Words with /ter/ = /tɚ/

Medial	IPA	Final	IPA
aftermath		blotter	
artery		clatter	
enterprise		janitor	
illiterate		equator	

Your List of /tɚ/ Words

Medial	IPA	Final	IPA

Words with /ther/ = /θɚ/

Medial	IPA	Final	IPA
authoring		author	
		panther	
		Luther	

Your List of /θɚ/ Words

Medial	IPA	Final	IPA

Words with /ver/ = /vɚ/

Medial	IPA	Final	IPA
beverage		ever	
favorite		lever	
oversight		savor	
several		endeavor	

Your List of /vɚ/ Words

Medial	IPA	Final	IPA

Words with /jer/ = /dʒɚ/

Medial	IPA	Final	IPA
dangerous		dodger	
injury		voyager	
gingerly		soldier	
majored		stranger	

Your List of /dʒɚ/ Words

Medial	IPA	Final	IPA

Words with /ser/ = /sɚ/

Medial	IPA	Final	IPA
grocery		chaser	
nursery		guesser	
glossary		placer	
sponsoring		compressor	

Your List of /sɚ/ Words

Medial	IPA	Final	IPA

Words with /yer/ = /jɚ/

Medial	IPA	Final	IPA
figurine		purer	
senior high		failure	
junior league		savior	
		refigure	

Your List of /jɚ/ Words

Medial	IPA	Final	IPA

Words with /zer/ = /zɚ/

Medial	IPA	Final	IPA
misery		cleanser	
reservoir		laser	
observing		composer	
reserved		incisor	

Your List of /zɚ/ Words

Medial	IPA	Final	IPA

Words with /zher/ = /ʒɚ/

Medial	IPA	Final	IPA
leisurely		closure	
measuring		Frazer	
treasury		composure	
pleasurable		foreclosure	

Your List of /ʒɚ/ Words

Medial	IPA	Final	IPA

Sentences with /ɚ/

1. The chemist was leisurely as he measured the compounds in his lab.
2. Misery loves company.
3. The composer found the song unfamiliar.
4. The stranger seemed dangerous.
5. Nevertheless this was her first oversight.
6. Who is authoring the book on international accents?
7. The pastor masterfully redirected the altercation during Sunday prayers.
8. The aspirin relived the pain and energized the player.
9. The caller said her son was allergic to certain types of cleaners.
10. The soccer player was seen staggering to the locker.

/ur/, /er/ = /ɝ/

1. Raise the central part of the tongue halfway toward the roof of the mouth (palate).

2. The tongue tip should be raised to rest just behind the front teeth (alveolar ridge).

3. The lips are rounded and open slightly.

4. Stress your "pose" to get it right and repeat multiple times till it feels comfortable.

5. Practice the sound in words and sentences.

Words with /ther/ = /ðɝ/

Medial	IPA	Final	IPA
bothering		gather	
lathering		slither	
otherwise		housemother	
tethering		together	

Your List of /ðɝ/ Words

Medial	IPA	Final	IPA

Recurring /ɚ/ within Words

burner	squanderer	easterner
turner	further	westerner
governor	gatherer	supervisor
emperor	liberator	experimenter

Your List of /ɚ/ Words

Practice Sentences with recurring /ɚ/

1. The governor was bothered by the easterner's attitude.
2. He spent so much that they called him "squanderer."
3. She moved so much that her friends called her a "wanderer."
4. The supervisor was upset about a burner that was destroyed in the lab.
5. Together we can make Sam look like an emperor.
6. Joe was promoted to his new job as a supervisor.
7. Jill could throw the ball further than Jim.
8. The weatherman was a westerner.
9. The liberator was beloved by his people.
10. The pilgrims were good hunters and gatherers.

6

Speech Sounds: Consonants

You have observed how the oral cavity changes shape when you prolong vowel sounds. You've also realized that production of vowel sounds is not a very visible process, so that more focused practice is required for your work with vowels. Now you are ready to put the vowels together with their counterparts, the consonants, to produce something meaningful: words. How are vowel sounds different from consonant sounds?

Consonants are the supportive speech sounds that combine with vowel sounds to form words (the word *consonant* means "sounding along with"). These speech sounds, or phonemes (the terms *sound* and *phoneme* are used interchangeably), are produced by the placement of the articulators (vocal organs) at different points of contact within the oral cavity. This causes various degrees of obstruction in the vocal tract. You are already aware that vowels are not produced as result of oral cavity obstruction. And you are also aware that the air is free flowing through the oral cavity without any obstacle in the case of vowels. However, the obstruction in the oral cavity by the articulators in turn blocks the air flow through the vocal tract producing different consonant sounds.

For example, let's compare how the two consonant sounds /p/ and /g/ are made. The phoneme /p/ is made when the air coming from the vocal tract is blocked completely by the lips and then released with a puff. Note that the obstruction for /p/ is at the *front* of the mouth. However, for voicing the phoneme /g/, the back of the tongue is raised to touch the posterior end of the hard palate to form the obstruction. The air passes through the vocal folds first, causing them to vibrate. The air is then released without a puff. Note that the obstruction for /g/ is at the *back* of the mouth.

Similarly, each of the consonants may be described in terms of point of obstruction and presence or absence of audible air flow. In this chapter, the consonants are grouped into simple categories based on the place and manner of obstruction, as determined by leading linguistic researchers and phoneticians. The presence or absence of vocal fold vibration, called *voicing*, is another very important feature that also assists in distinguishing among the consonant sounds. As you read through the descriptions within each of the categories, visualize the articulators within your mouth and identify their points of contact in the oral cavity in order to achieve correct pronunciation.

Before we proceed to the details of consonant classification, let's return to the phonetic symbols. Similar to the vowels, each of the consonants also has a phonetic symbol in the International Phonetic Alphabet format (IPA). The IPA phonetic symbols for the consonants are used throughout this chapter. Keep in mind that there are no shortcuts to learning the phonetic symbols—they must be *memorized*. English/phonetic consonant symbol comparisons are summarized in a Consonant Legend table at the end of this chapter.

Consonant Classification

The consonants traditionally are classified by three basic features:

- place of articulation
- manner of articulation
- voicing

Understanding how each of these features is involved in creating the consonant sounds is essential. As you will explore in the worksheet exercises, the difference between two consonants may be quite subtle, with only a slight variation in just one of the features. The consonants are accurately recognized by using all three features.

Place of Articulation

Place of articulation refers to the *position* at which the articulators contact and *where* the closure or narrowing of the vocal tract takes place to form the speech sounds. Once you identify the contact position of the articulators for a specific consonant and place them correctly, you will improve production of your consonant sounds.

Some consonants are recognizable through visual cues observed as the sound is produced by the speaker. For example, when we observe a speaker press the lips together, we can guess that the sound may be a /p/, /b/, or /m/. *Looking at the speaker's mouth* to observe certain maneuvers in speech production can be very helpful in understanding unfamiliar words or accents.

How does this help with accent management? Knowing where the points of contact for the various articulators are for each of the speech consonants makes it easier to modify the resulting sound in your pronunciation. Although it may seem that you are exaggerating your speech production, with consistent practice the modification will come naturally within conversation.

Table 6–1 illustrates the list of consonants showing minimal or no contact up to maximum or complete contact with the articulators, starting from the back of the mouth to the front. Notice that the contact increases and the positions vary for the different consonants of the English language.

Manner of Articulation

Manner of articulation refers to the *degree of narrowing* of the vocal tract that obstructs the air flow. This feature of consonants is more complex, less visual, and hence more difficult to recognize. The narrowing or obstruction that occurs with production of each consonant sound varies depending on whether the point of contact is at the front (lips), middle, (palate), or back (velum) of the mouth. With each location, different degrees of narrowing or obstruction result, with either partial or complete block of the air flow. Use of different articulators combined with various degrees of obstruction produces the different consonant sounds.

Table 6–1. Consonants Grouped by Type of Contact with Articulators

/h/	Minimal or no contact
/k, g, ŋ/	Back of the tongue raises up to touch the soft palate
/j, ʧ, ʃ, dʒ, ʒ, r/	Tongue blade (sides) touches inner surfaces of the molars on both sides of the mouth
/t, d, n, s, z, l/	Tongue tip strokes the ridge just behind the front teeth
/ð, θ/	Tongue tip sticks out through the front teeth
/p, b, m/	Lips pressed together
/w/	Lips pulled together in a "pucker" position and rounded

For example, when you utter the /h/ sound, the air from your lungs flows freely out of your mouth. Neither your tongue nor your lips interrupt the flow. However, for sounds like /p/ or /m/, the lips interrupt the air flow by blocking the flow as they press together or are released in a puff. Similarly, for the production of sounds like /t/ or /s/, the tongue tip touches the alveolar ridge behind the teeth to create an interruption, followed by partial release of air.

The only way to study the manner of articulation is by tactile cues or awareness by touch. Once the correct position or place of articulation is set, stop to get a "feel" for the point of contact. This will identify the exact spot and help you to return to that same spot each time you produce the consonant.

For example, compare the phonemes /t/ and /d/. The tongue tip for /t/ is closer to the alveolar ridge (behind the front teeth), but the point of contact for /d/ is farther from the ridge and closer to the middle of the hard palate (roof of the mouth). Once you "feel" the point of contact, memorize it and practice positioning the tongue tip till it feels comfortable.

If you are working with a speech therapist, he or she can provide you with immediate feedback to help you learn how to produce the correct consonant sound during a session. Sometimes a tactile cue—a touch or other stimulus—can be supplied by the therapist. For example, a tongue depressor can be used to touch the point of contact in your mouth to help give you a sensation of articulator placement.

However, home practice requires the use of a mirror to visually record your responses to the practice drills. The mirror will give you the feedback when a speech therapist is not present. Still, try to begin with the correct placement demonstrated by a professional speech therapist before you begin your home practice in earnest. In addition, listen carefully to the sound each consonant makes, while watching for the correct point of placement—as sounds like /t/ and /d/ may have the same point of placement but differ in other properties such as air release (aspiration). Once you become familiar with the point of contact necessary for the production of each of the speech sounds, practice drills become easy. You will be able to correct your home practice and record your progress.

Consonant Groupings

There are 24 different consonant sounds grouped into five different categories based on air flow. The entire set of consonants categorized by the manner of articulation is listed in Table 6–2. Place your hand in front of your mouth and try saying the consonant sounds out loud as you go down the list. You can feel the air flow on your hand indicating presence or absence of air release.

Voicing

Voicing is critical to the clarity of spoken English and affects accent. This speech sound property refers to the movements of the vocal folds (your "vocal cords"), termed *vocal fold vibration* by speech-language professionals. The vocal folds vibrate when air passes through them. These vibrations are important determinants of articulation along with the place and manner of articulation. You can feel the vocal fold vibration when you *place a hand on your throat*. This is an excellent way to practice to make sure you producing correct voicing.

The consonants of the English language can be grouped according to the presence or absence of vocal fold vibration:

- *Voiced consonants*: There is significant vocal fold vibration. /w, m, v, ð, n, l, j, r, ŋ, z, ʒ, dʒ, b, d, g/
- *Voiceless consonants*: Vocal fold vibration does not occur. /f, θ, h, s, tʃ, ʃ, p, t, k/

Most speech therapists recommend practicing these sounds in pairs to identify the presence or absence of voicing. For example, /p/ and /b/ may be practiced alternately. Place your hand on your throat and say /p/ and then /b/; feel the differences in voicing—/p/ is voiceless, /b/ is voiced. Similarly, other pairs are /t/ and /d/, /m/ and /n/, /ð/ and /θ/, and /tʃ/ and /dʒ/. Practice with these pairs may be benefited by using a tactile or touch cue (with the hand).

Place and manner of articulation, along with voicing, make up the traditional classification system of consonant sounds. For example, /p/ can be described as speech sound produced by using both lips (place = lips), has air released with a puff (manner = blocked air flow), and has no vocal fold vibration (voiceless). Similarly, all conso-

Table 6–2. Consonants Grouped by Airflow

Noisy Airflow Continuous air flow with partial closure and release through a narrow cavities of the articulators: **fricatives**	/f, v, ð, θ, s, z, ʃ, ʒ/
Free Airflow Continuous air released through mouth; articulator moves from one position to another: **glides**	/w, l, j, r, h/
Air flow through the nose: **nasals**	/m, n, ŋ/
Blocked Airflow Air flow blocked by the articulators and released with a puff: **stops**	/p, b, t, d, k, g/
Air is completely blocked by articulator position and then vocal tract partially opens to allow restricted air flow through a narrow opening: **affricates**	/tʃ, dʒ/

nant sounds can be described using these three features.

Familiarizing yourself with these three features will help you understand the art of speech sound production and its effects on correcting your accent. Other features that help classify speech sounds are used by speech pathologists and researchers in the fields of linguistics and phonetics; these are beyond the scope of this text.

Phonetic versus Alphabetic Consonant Sounds

Even though the process of speech sound production is more visible with consonants than with vowels, and although consonant sounds have fewer spelling variations compared with vowels, use of the phonetic fonts to distinguish between the phonemes is essential. For example, to differentiate between ch in "**ch**at" versus ch in "**ch**aracter" (the /k/ sound) or in "**ch**ef" (the /sh/ sound), the use of the IPA symbols—/ʃ/ for the /sh/

sound in "chef" versus /tʃ/ for the standard /ch/ in "chat"—makes the correct pronunciation perfectly clear.

Refer to Table 6–3 comparing English and phonetic (IPA) symbols with example words. The symbols *must* be memorized for phonetic transcription practice (see Chapter 4).

Summary

Consonants are produced by means of various degrees of obstruction created by the placement of articulators. Place, manner, and voicing all are important components of consonant production. The use of phonetic symbols to decipher spelling variations is vital for correct pronunciation, as you have noticed with phonetic transcription. The symbols *must* be memorized for phonetic transcription practice (see Chapter 4).

Worksheet 6–1 provides practice words and sentences and phonetic transcription exercises for all of the consonant speech sounds.

Table 6–3. Consonants Compared by English and Phonetic Symbols

Consonant Legend			
Speech Sound	**IPA**	**IPA in Words**	**English Spelling**
p	p	pæn	pan
b	b	bæn	ban
k	k	kɪt, kejɔs	kit, chaos
g	g	gæm	game
th	θ	θɪnk	think
dh	ð	ðer	there
t	t	tem	tame
d	d	dɪm	dim
s	s	sæl, saɪt	sale, cite
z	z	zu	zoo
ch	tʃ	tʃɪp	chip
dz	dʒ	dʒɑr	jar
sh	ʃ	ʃɨp, ʃɛf	sheep, chef
zh	ʒ	trɛʒɚr	treasure
m	m	maʊs	mouse
n	n	naɪn	nine
ng	ŋ	θɪŋ	thing
h	h	hɑp	hop
l	l	laɪk	like
f	f	fɪt	feet
r	r	rum	room
v	v	vez	vase
w	w	wɪt	wit
ya	j	jɑŋ	young

WORKSHEET 6

Consonant Practice

Instructions

1. Consonant speech sounds are divided into the following patterns of units for targeted practice:
   - Minimal pairs (examples: /k/ and /g/, /m/ and /n/)
   - Other sounds (example: /ing/)
   - Blends (examples: sl, sm, br)

2. Consonant Sounds are divided according to their position within words:
   - Exceptions
   - Initial (phoneme in the beginning of the word)
   - Medial (phoneme in the middle of the word)
   - Final (phoneme at the end of the word)

3. The practice words are grouped according to graded difficulty (mono or disyllabic versus multisyllabic); the word lists are followed by practice sentences.

4. Blank columns are provided for phonetic transcription (IPA), and for creating your own lists of words for practice.

5. Use the following Consonant Legend table of IPA symbols to identify the correct pronunciation.

6. Challenge yourself by reusing the worksheets and adding new vocabulary words for pronunciation practice.

Consonant Legend			
Speech Sound	**IPA**	**IPA in Words**	**English Spelling**
p	p	p æ n	pan
b	b	b æ n	ban
k	k	k ɪ t, k e j ɔ s	kit, chaos
g	g	g æ m	game
th	θ	θ ɪ n k	think
dh	ð	ð e r	there
t	t	t e m	tame
d	d	d ɪ m	dim
s	s	s æ l, s aɪ t	sale, cite
z	z	z u	zoo
ch	tʃ	tʃ ɪ p	chip
dz	dʒ	dʒ ɑ r	jar
sh	ʃ	ʃ ɨ p, ʃ ɛ f	sheep, chef
zh	ʒ	t r ɛ ʒ ə r	treasure
m	m	m aʊ s	mouse
n	n	n aɪ n	nine
ng	ŋ	θ ɪ ŋ	thing
h	h	h ɑ p	hop
l	l	l aɪ k	like
f	f	f ɪ t	feet
r	r	r u m	room
v	v	v e z	vase
w	w	w ɪ t	wit
ya	j	j ɑ ŋ	young

Instructions:

1. Place your hand on your throat. Feel for the bony protrusion of your voice box and rest your fingers on the surrounding area.

2. Say /**k**/ and then /**g**/ slowly, multiple times, and feel the different sensation in your throat. You should notice minimal feeling while saying /**k**/ and a significant vibration while saying /**g**/.

3. Practice other sound pairs: /p/ and /b/, /t/ and /d/, /s/ and /z/, /f/ and /v/, and so on.

4. Observe the positions of the articulators within the vocal tract and the presence or absence of air flow/release.

5. Repeat the consonant sounds multiple times until you feel comfortable with the place and manner of articulation and the voicing of each sound.

6. Proceed to the word lists for practice.

Minimal Pairs /k/ and /g/

/k/ as in "kite" and "cane"

1. Start with raising the back of your tongue to touch the back of the mouth (velum). This blocks the breath stream.

2. Pull away the back of your tongue in a quick motion to release a burst of air as you say /**k**/. This is referred to as aspiration.

3. Place a hand on your throat—you have to *stop* voicing here to clearly say /**k**/.

4. Stress your "pose" to get it right and repeat multiple times until it feels comfortable.

5. Practice each sound in the initial, medial, and final positions within words.

6. Graduate to sentences after completing the word isolation drills.

7. Write each word in IPA format for before pronunciation practice.

Exceptions for /k/ Speech Sound

English Spelling	IPA	English Spelling	IPA
ache		evoke	
headache		plaque	
Bach		Luke	
beefcakes		oblique	
mandrake		stake	

/k/ Sound Appearing Twice within Words

English Spelling	IPA	English Spelling	IPA
cucumber		Kentucky	
caretaker		contradict	
cracker		cataract	
cookie		counteract	
coconut		kayaking	

Words with /k/ in Initial, Medial, and Final Positions

Initial	IPA	Medial	IPA	Final	IPA
king		beaker		weak	
kin		baking		week	
Kenneth		racket		tick	
Kurt		sicken		peck	
Kyle		awaken		hawk	

Your List of /k/ Words

Initial	IPA	Medial	IPA	Final	IPA

*Words with /**k**/ sound with the letter **c** in Initial, Medial, and Final Positions*

Initial	IPA	Medial	IPA	Final	IPA
cab		accord		basic	
come		account		attic	
calm		bacon		attack	
came		boycott		clinic	
coax		acne		drastic	

*Your List of /**k**/ Words with the letter **c**￼*

Initial	IPA	Medial	IPA	Final	IPA

*Multisyllable Words with /**k**/ Sound in the Initial, Medial and Final Positions*

Initial	IPA	Medial	IPA	Final	IPA
kangaroo		acknowledge		broomstick	
kayaking		awakened		boardwalk	
keyboard		pocket watch		flapjack	
kerosene		ukulele		shamrock	
kindergarten		walking shoes		livestock	

*Your List of Multisyllable /**k**/ Words*

Initial	IPA	Medial	IPA	Final	IPA

*Multisyllable Words with /k/ Sound with the letter **c** in Initial, Medial, and Final Positions*

Initial	IPA	Medial	IPA	Final	IPA
capture		academy		graphic	
Cambodia		accordion		frolic	
catastrophe		bicarbonate		Pontiac	
coalition		despicable		dramatic	
carnivorous		domesticate		optimistic	

*Your List of Multisyllable /k/ Words with the letter **c***

Initial	IPA	Medial	IPA	Final	IPA

/g/ as in "gate"

1. Start with raising the back of your tongue to touch the back of the mouth (velum). This blocks the breath stream—no aspiration or air is released.

2. Pull away the back of your tongue in a quick motion as you make the /g/ sound.

3. Place a hand on your throat—you have to *feel* voicing here to clearly say /g/.

4. Stress your "pose" to get it right and repeat multiple times until it feels comfortable.

5. Practice each sound in the initial, medial. and final positions within words

6. Graduate to sentences after completing the word isolation drills.

7. Write each word in IPA format before pronunciation practice.

Exceptions for /g/

English Spelling	IPA	English Spelling	IPA
fatigue		colleague	
intrigue		synagogue	
vague		travelogue	
vogue		monologue	
Hague		Prague	

Words with /g/ as in "gate" and /dʒ/ as in "jar" and "age"

English Spelling	IPA	English Spelling	IPA
bondage		gauge	
postage		garage	
wreckage		gigantic	
ageless		ginger	
digest		geography	

Words with /g/ in Initial, Medial, and Final Positions

Initial	IPA	Medial	IPA	Final	IPA
gap		august		bag	
game		again		twig	
gait		beggar		beg	
gauze		bigot		bog	
gear		bygones		brag	

Your List of /g/ Words

Initial	IPA	Medial	IPA	Final	IPA

Multisyllable Words with /g/ in Initial Medial and Final Positions

Initial	IPA	Medial	IPA	Final	IPA
gadget		agonize		bear hug	
gallop		arrogance		bedbug	
gamble		begonia		bean bag	
garage		beginning		guide dog	
gazelle		category		hedgehog	

Your List of Multisyllable /g/ Words

Initial	IPA	Medial	IPA	Final	IPA

Sentences with /k/ and /g/

Identify the presence and absence of *aspiration* or *air release* to isolate the "correct" pronunciation of /k/ and /g/ in the following sentences.

1. Carol's cucumber salad was delicious.
2. The committee came to an agreement, comfortable for all concerned.
3. Callie likes coconut cookies.
4. She always carried her brown bag lunch with her.
5. The children had fun with the three-legged race at the Carnegie Fair.
6. There was a gigantic statue of a giraffe at Gideon's house.
7. Colleen's report captured the essence of Connecticut.
8. Eric made a dramatic entrance at the Cowan's party.
9. It was a gamble to buy the headgear at that store.
10. The antique racquet was crucial to Carla's Sixties Sports party.
11. It was beginner's luck that she won all that money gambling!
12. Do not antagonize the officer at the Pentagon.
13. The academy offered courses in economics and mathematics.
14. Agonizing over small issues magnifies it threefold.

15. Use paper or cloth bags for your groceries.

16. Peg is snug as a bug in a rug.

17. Ken likes kickball and Carla likes kayaking.

18. Arrogance is usually a big cause for one's downfall.

19. Logan is practicing as a legal secretary in Hugo's office.

20. Let's go backpacking across Africa.

Minimal Pairs /p/ and /b/

/p/ as in "park"

The /p/ sound requires aspiration. So "park" is pronounced /p(h)ark/, where the (h) denotes presence of aspiration.

1. Start with pressing your lips together to block the air stream.

2. Release your lips with a burst of air (aspiration) to /a/ position.

3. Your lips rest in an oval position as you finish producing the sound /p(h)a/.

4. Place a hand on your throat—you have to *stop* voicing here to clearly say /4/.

5. Stress your "pose" to get it right and repeat multiple times until it feels comfortable.

6. Practice each sound in the initial, medial, and final positions within words.

7. Graduate to sentences after completing the word isolation drills.

Exceptions: /p/ appearing Twice within Words

English Spelling	IPA	English Spelling	IPA	English Spelling	IPA
pepper		pumpernickel		paperboy	
paper		perpendicular		pampered	
peppercorns		paperback		pop-up	
pumpkin		puppet		Paprika	
peppermint		perception		paperweight	

*Words with the letters **pe** for Final /**p**/ Sound*

English Spelling	IPA	English Spelling	IPA	English Spelling	IPA
coupe		scrape		Slope	
crepe		snipe		Mope	
cantaloupe		fire escape		horoscope	
envelope		periscope		prototype	
semi-ripe		audiotape		cinemascope	

*Words with /**p**/ in Initial, Medial, and Final Positions*

Initial	IPA	Medial	IPA	Final	IPA
padlock		appeared		backdrop	
pinched		depot		closeup	
pierce		flapjack		postop	
Pierre		scrapbook		turnip	
Peru		upgrade		swap	

*Your List of /**p**/ Words*

Initial	IPA	Medial	IPA	Final	IPA

*Multisyllable Words with /**p**/ in Initial, Medial and Final Positions*

Initial	IPA	Medial	IPA	Final	IPA
Patricia		haphazard		buttercup	
Pearl Harbor		grasshopper		censorship	
Poughkeepsie		operation		coffee-cup	
performance		recapping		fellowship	
picturesque		recapitulate		workshop	

Your List of Multisyllable /p/ Words

Initial	IPA	Medial	IPA	Final	IPA

/b/ as in "bay"

1. Start with pressing your lips together to block the air stream.
2. Release your lips without a burst of air to /a/ position (no aspiration).
3. Your lips rest in an oval position as you finish producing the sound /ba/.
4. Place a hand on your throat to *feel* voicing in that area, to clearly say /**b**/.
5. Stress your "pose" to get it right and repeat multiple times until it feels comfortable.
6. Practice each sound in the initial, medial and final positions within words
7. Graduate to sentences after completing the word isolation drills.

Exceptions: /b/ Appearing Twice Within Words

English Spelling	IPA	English Spelling	IPA	English Spelling	IPA
babble		Barbara		bubble	
baboon		Bible		bumblebee	
baby		Big Bird		barbaric	
Bobby		bobcat		blueberry	
barber		bobsled		Big Ben	

/b/ Sound Spelled with the letters be

English Spelling	IPA	English Spelling	IPA	English Spelling	IPA
cube		tube		prescribe	
globe		strobe		inscribe	
tribe		ascribe		subscribe	
lube		describe		test-tube	
vibe		transcribe		wardrobe	

Words with /b/ in Initial, Medial, and Final Positions

Initial	IPA	Medial	IPA	Final	IPA
bombard		subway		bob	
borrow		tubing		rob	
burden		tugboat		crab	
bushel		bobbin		hub	
bypass		subject		dab	

Your List of /b/ Words

Initial	IPA	Medial	IPA	Final	IPA

Multisyllable Words with /b/ in the Initial Medial and Final Positions

Initial	IPA	Medial	IPA	Final	IPA
botanical		submarine		snow job	
biologist		disability		photo lab	
bucketful		observatory		picture tube	
bulletin		suburbanite		hubbub	
bungalow		website		doorknob	

Your List of Multisyllable /b/ Words

Initial	IPA	Medial	IPA	Final	IPA

Sentences with /p/ and /b/

Identify the presence or absence of *aspiration* or *air release* to isolate the "correct" pronunciation in the following sentences.

1. The principal called Bobby to his office.
2. Baby Barbara was just starting to babble.
3. Pamela had a craving for papaya and a Popsicle.
4. Bert went to his barber on a busy afternoon.
5. She would like some popcorn and pumpernickel bread.
6. He bribed his barber into letting him use his beach house.
7. Do you like pepper on your pizza?
8. Blake baked a banana cake for Bobby and Bert.
9. The puppet show was perceived as pretentious.
10. Bernice was set with her wardrobe for the school year.
11. Patricia has piano lessons with Mr. Brown.
12. Blanche barbecued vegetable burgers for the Benson's family.
13. Piper made pumpkin pie for the party.
14. Peter took pain pills before his kickball game.
15. The doorknob of the bathroom needs to be replaced.
16. Baby Pam was pampered with popcorn and popsicles by her grandmother.
17. Billions of people petitioned against the new rules.
18. She bought new pearls for the beauty pageant.
19. Paul was late for his appointment at the photo shoot.
20. Don't eavesdrop on people's conversations.

Minimal Pairs /tʃ/ and /dʒ/

/tʃ/ as in "choo-choo train"

1. Raise the *tongue tip* and place it flat right behind your front teeth (alveolar ridge).
2. Apply some pressure as you rest the tongue tip on the ridge behind the teeth.
3. Allow the *sides* of the tongue to touch the *side teeth* to block the air flow.
4. Keep your mouth slightly puckered and open.
5. Start with the upper and lower teeth resting against each other.
6. Build up air pressure and release explosively.
7. Notice how the mouth opens and the tongue moves back (sounds like "choo-choo train").
8. Place a hand on your throat—you have to *stop* voicing here to clearly say /tʃ/.
9. Stress your "pose" to get it right and repeat multiple times until it feels comfortable.
10. Practice each sound in the initial, medial, and final positions within words.
11. Graduate to sentences after performing the word isolation drills.

Exceptions for /tʃ/ Sound

Write each word in IPA format for before pronunciation practice.

English Spelling	IPA	English Spelling	IPA
fracture		punctuate	
gesture		mutual	
cello		natural	
venture		fistula	
rapture		situate	

Words with /tʃ/ in Initial, Medial, and Final Positions

Initial	IPA	Medial	IPA	Final	IPA
chain		blue cheese		clutch	
charter		catching		clench	
chapped		chitchat		Mitch	
Charlie		ketchup		Blanche	
Charleston		notches		French	

Your List of /tʃ/ Words

Initial	IPA	Medial	IPA	Final	IPA

Multisyllable Words with /tʃ/ in Initial, Medial and Final Positions

Initial	IPA	Medial	IPA	Final	IPA
checkerboard		anchovy		Attach	
checkmate		patchwork		Bewitch	
chimney		recharge		cross stitch	
chopsticks		pitch-black		homestretch	
churchyard		touchdown		hopscotch	

Your List of Multisyllable /tʃ/ Words

Initial	IPA	Medial	IPA	Final	IPA

/dʒ/ as in "jump"

1. *Raise* the *tongue tip* and place it flat right behind your front teeth (alveolar ridge).

2. Apply some pressure as you rest the tongue tip on the ridge behind the teeth.

3. Allow the *sides* of your tongue to touch the *side teeth* to block the air flow.

4. Keep your lips slightly puckered and and your mouth open.

5. Start with the upper and lower teeth resting against each other.

6. Build up air pressure and release explosively.

7. Notice how the mouth opens and the tongue moves back.

8. Place a hand on your throat—you have to *feel* voicing here to clearly say /dʒ/.

9. Stress your "pose" to get it right and repeat multiple times until it feels comfortable.

10. Practice each sound in the initial, medial, and final positions within words

11. Graduate to sentences after completing the word isolation drills.

*Exception: Words with the letter **g** as /dʒ/ Sound in Initial, Medial, and Final Positions*

Initial	IPA	Medial	IPA	Final	IPA
gel		eligible		age	
gem		agent		edge	
gene		hedges		gauge	
ginger		eulogy		cartridge	
gypsy		pledging		wreckage	

*Your List of letter **g** Words with /dʒ/ Sound*

Initial	IPA	Medial	IPA	Final	IPA

*Words with /**dʒ**/ Sound in Initial, Medial, and Final Positions*

Initial	IPA	Medial	IPA	Final	IPA
Jacob		adjourn		Taj	
Jack		adjunct		Raj	
Jean		adjust		Bajaj	
Jaguar		adjoin			
jockey		adjacent			

*Your List of Words with /**dʒ**/ Sound*

Initial	IPA	Medial	IPA	Final	IPA

*Multisyllable Words with /**dʒ**/ Sound in Initial, Medial, and Final Positions*

Initial	IPA	Medial	IPA	Final	IPA
ginseng		agitation		Anchorage	
gigantic		fugitive		scrounge	
jaundice		suggestion		impinge	
jealous		tragically		rearrange	
joyous		ejection		brokerage	

*Your List of Multisyllable /**dʒ**/ Words*

Initial	IPA	Medial	IPA	Final	IPA

Sentences with /tʃ/ and /dʒ/

1. Mitch wants to go to Myrtle Beach this summer
2. Charles carries his checkbook in his briefcase.
3. Jake was asked to change his style and the language of his presentation.
4. Jack majored in journalism at his junior college.
5. The cheerleaders from Cherryville chatted on the charter bus.
6. The management structure promoted autocratic style.
7. Roger delivered an excellent eulogy.
8. Ryan thought it was magical to watch the Dodgers game.
9. He was an amateur journalist with a charming attitude.
10. Did you check the dosage chart today?
11. Do you like ginseng tea?
12. It is a challenge to rearrange someone else's schedule.
13. Jean was jealous of Jan's promotion and was also discouraged by the layoffs.
14. Jason and Jonathan went to Jakarta in January.
15. Juniper and Jupiter were funny names for pets.
16. China and Japan won most of the medals in gymnastics.
17. The Chamber of Commerce is on Church Street.
18. Who is making the next batch of chocolate chip cookies?
19. Patch was the best sheep dog at the county fair.
20. Listen to Peg Thatcher calling out the lotto numbers for a match.

Minimal Pairs /m/ and /n/

/m/ as in "may"

1. Start with puckering your lips.
2. Say /a/ as you open up your lips to /a/ position.
3. Your lips rest in an oval position as you finish producing the sound /ma/.
4. Place a hand on your throat—you have to *stop* voicing here to clearly say /m/.
5. Stress your "pose" to get it right and repeat multiple times until it feels comfortable.
6. Practice each sound in the initial, medial, and final positions within words.
7. Graduate to sentences after completing the word isolation drills.

*Exceptions: Words with /**m**/ in Final Position*

-m	IPA	-me	IPA	-ym	IPA
mayhem		slime		pseudonym	
random		thyme		paradigm	
sternum		rhyme		antonym	
modem		phoneme		homonym	

-lm	IPA	-sm	IPA
Stockholm		chasm	
calm		neoplasm	
palm		spasm	
realm		enthusiasm	

*Words with /**m**/ in Initial, Medial, and Final Positions*

Initial	IPA	Medial	IPA	Final	IPA
madness		dome		cram	
morbid		comet		farm	
major		mummy		stream	
might		shimmy		gloom	
Morton		blooming		tram	

*Your List of /**m**/ Words*

Initial	IPA	Medial	IPA	Final	IPA

*Multisyllable Words with /**m**/ in Initial, Medial and Final Positions*

Initial	IPA	Medial	IPA	Final	IPA
marquis		squirming		forearm	
meteorite		rummage		theorem	
mourning		summoned		aquarium	
mistletoe		tombstone		auditorium	
mohair		tumbling		sour cream	

*Your List of Multisyllable /**m**/ Words*

Initial	IPA	Medial	IPA	Final	IPA

/n/ as in "nose"

1. Start with puckering your lips.
2. Say /a/ as you open up your lips to /a/ position.
3. Your lips rest in an oval position as you finish producing the sound /**na**/.
4. Place a hand on your throat—you have to *stop* voicing here to clearly say /**n**/.
5. Stress your "pose" to get it right and repeat multiple times until it feels comfortable.
6. Practice each sound in the initial, medial, and final positions within words.
7. Graduate to sentences after performing the word isolation drills.

Exceptions: Words with /n/ in Final Position

/n/	IPA	/rn/	IPA	/yn/	IPA
African		scorn		Jaclyn	
patrolman		stern		Lynn	
woman		torn		Evelyn	
skeleton		warn		Wynn	
indecision		sworn		Roslyn	

/ne/	IPA	/wn/	IPA	/mn/	IPA
done		blown		damn	
Verne		yawn		solemn	
humane		Shawn		column	
cologne		overgrown			
hydroplane		clown			

Words with /n/ in Initial, Medial, and Final Positions

Initial	IPA	Medial	IPA	Final	IPA
nap		mundane		mean	
neat		sundown		terrain	
nibble		shindig		resin	
noble		sonnet		raisin	
nut		running		tailspin	

Your List of /n/ Words

Initial	IPA	Medial	IPA	Final	IPA

Multisyllable Words with /n/ in Initial, Medial and Final Position

Initial	IPA	Medial	IPA	Final	IPA
Nebraska		anatomy		remission	
narcissistic		monastery		triathlon	
nitrogen		inaudible		nomination	
neonatal		Rangoon		superhuman	
nourishment		signing		phenomenon	

Your List of Multisyllable Words with /n/

Initial	IPA	Medial	IPA	Final	IPA

Sentences with /m/ and /n/

1. The German highway system is called autobahn.
2. The drummer was murmuring to himself.
3. Does Norma want to play a mermaid in the show?
4. As a journalist, you can utilize the freedom of speech.
5. Mr. Smith explained his problem animatedly.
6. Anna is an elementary school teacher.
7. Children of each generation turn into amazing and accomplished adults.
8. Samantha had a bad reaction to poison ivy.
9. Norman was inarticulate and disorganized at the board meeting.
10. Kenneth and Mona make a good management team.
11. Where is the manual for the manufacturing guidelines?
12. Janet was honored for her magnificent contribution to the project.
13. Enid and Marla coordinated the March Madness Day in their development.
14. Parental involvement is very important in every child's growth.
15. Mara repented not taking the management position offered to her by the previous company.

16. The drafts were sent to the builders and a tentative date for the meeting is set.

17. She seemed confident and energetic before the performance.

18. Silence of golden.

19. Martha and Nina went snowboarding on Wednesday.

20. The accommodations for the tournament were arranged by the school.

Minimal Pairs /s/ and /z/

/s/ as in "hiss"

1. Raise the tip of your tongue to nearly contact the ridge behind your upper teeth.

2. Position the sides of the tongue to come in contact with the inner surfaces of the upper teeth.

3. This creates a small fold along the midline of the tongue.

4. Air flow is directed through this fold to make the /s/ sound. This produces a noisy hissing sound.

5. Place a hand on your throat—you have to *stop* voicing here to say /s/.

6. Stress your "pose" to get it right and repeat multiple times until it feels comfortable.

7. Practice each sound in the initial, medial, and final positions within words.

8. Graduate to sentences after completing the word isolation drills.

Exceptions for /s/ sound

1. The letter **s** is pronounced as /z/ when it indicates a voiced plural.

Final	IPA	Final	IPA
draws		rays	
chooses		sees	
crows		spies	
days		toys	

Other examples of /s/ as /z/ in plural endings:

/bz/	IPA	/dz/	IPA	/ldz/	IPA
labs		adds		builds	
ribs		beads		colds	
bathrobes		codes		folds	
doorknobs		crowds		guilds	

/gz/	IPA	/lz/	IPA	/mz/	IPA	/nz/	IPA
lags		ails		beams		balloons	
legs		bails		dooms		clowns	
tags		bells		bums		drains	
rugs		bowls		calms		buttons	

/rz/	IPA	/vz/	IPA	/wz/	IPA
fairs		calves		bows	
chairs		caves		stows	
floors		cloves		cows	
hears		dives		eyebrows	

2. Plural marker is pronounced /ez/ (separate syllable) when attached to a noun or verb with sound endings of /s/, as in house = houses; /ch/, as in ditch = ditches; and /dz/, as in lunge = lunges.

ez			
Final	**IPA**	**Final**	**IPA**
hoses		twitches	
classes		plunges	
noses		sledges	
raises		stitches	

3. /s/ Sound Pronounced as /**z**/ in Medial Position

Medial	IPA	Medial	IPA	Medial	IPA
asthma		closes		business	
easier		cleanser		Caesar	
Boise		easel		laser	

Recurring /s/ Sounds within Words

English Spelling	IPA	English Spelling	IPA	English Spelling	IPA
circus		subside		insecticide	
license		succeed		narcissist	
recess		incense		satisfaction	
scentless		sickness		susceptible	
sequence		sensible		trespassing	

Your List of Words with Recurring /s/

English Spelling	IPA	English Spelling	IPA	English Spelling	IPA

Words with /s/ in Initial, Medial, and Final Positions

Initial	IPA	Medial	IPA	Final	IPA
serve		gossip		dress	
setting		guessing		loose	
seed		hissing		floss	
Sacramento		fussing		basis	
saddened		astringent		cross	

Your List of /s/ Words

Initial	IPA	Medial	IPA	Final	IPA

*Words with /s/ Sound with the letters **c** or **ce** in Initial, Medial, and Final Positions*

Initial	IPA	Medial	IPA	Final	IPA
cement		precinct		race	
cellular		faucet		brace	
cellophane		recede		sacrifice	
centennial		success		service	
century		precede		enhance	

*Your List of /s/ Words with a **c** or **ce***

Initial	IPA	Medial	IPA	Final	IPA

Multisyllable Words with /s/ in Initial, Medial, and Final Positions

Initial	IPA	Medial	IPA	Final	IPA
century		assortment		business	
surgeon		bicycle		bypass	
surprise		casino		usefulness	
certainly		casserole		diabetes	
cinnamon		classical		caboose	

Your List of Multisyllable /s/ Words

Initial	IPA	Medial	IPA	Final	IPA

/z/ as in "buzzing bee"

1. Raise the tip of your tongue to nearly contact the ridge behind your upper teeth.
2. Place the sides of the tongue come in contact with the inner surfaces of the upper teeth.
3. This creates a small fold along the midline of the tongue.
4. Air flow is directed through this fold to make the /z/ sound. This produces a noisy hissing sound.
5. Place a hand on your throat—you have to feel the voicing here to say /z/.
6. Stress your "pose" to get it right and repeat multiple times until it feels comfortable.
7. Practice each sound in the initial, medial, and final positions within words.
8. Graduate to sentences after completing the word isolation drills.

Exception: /x/ in Medial Position Pronounced as /gz/

/gz/ medial	IPA	/gz/ medial	IPA
exhibit		exasperation	
Exotic		exhaustion	
exaggerate		exertion	
executive		examination	
exemplary		exhilaration	

Words with /z/ in Initial, Medial, and Final Positions

Initial	IPA	Medial	IPA	Final	IPA
zillion		sizing		quiz	
zoom lens		gazelle		size	
zooming		sneezing		seize	
Zurich		hazard		sneeze	
zipper		seized		snooze	

Your List of /z/ Words

Initial	IPA	Medial	IPA	Final	IPA

Multisyllable Words with /z/ in Initial, Medial and Final Positions

Initial	IPA	Medial	IPA	Final	IPA
czarina		easement		baptize	
xylophone		jasmine		bulldoze	
zebra fish		Kansas City		analyze	
zeppelin		nosebleed		paralyze	
zestfully		reasoning		criticize	

Your List of Multisyllable /z/ Words

Initial	IPA	Medial	IPA	Final	IPA

Sentences with /s/ and /z/

1. Is it safe to go cycling through these woods?
2. She sounds like she can solve this problem.
3. Cinderella celebrated her sixteenth birthday.
4. Zoë lives in Boise, Idaho.
5. Zach had a severe case of asthma.
6. There was no trace of juice spills on this floor.
7. Curtis went to Dallas with Doris on Saturday.
8. Alice was cautious not to confess to spying on her friend.
9. What are you doing there, down on your hands and knees?
10. Zelda gave her baby's clothes away.
11. Sally went to Central Park to celebrate her 60th birthday.
12. Alison wanted to be an ambitious actress.
13. He had to submit his project by Saturday.
14. The message said to meet Cynthia at the massage parlor.
15. Did you make a deposit on Thursday?
16. Mozart was a famous composer and a musician.
17. The reasoning behind last week's disaster is beyond comprehension.
18. Excuse me for emphasizing the obvious.
19. Eunice and Harris went to the movies with Iris and Janice.
20. Denzel had a meeting in Kansas City on Wednesday.

Minimal Pairs /ʃ/ and /ʒ/

/ʃ/ as in "sheep"

1. Raise the tip of your tongue toward the roof of your mouth, behind the upper teeth.
2. Position the sides of the tongue to come in contact with the inner surfaces of the upper teeth.
3. This creates a small groove along the midline of the tongue.
4. Air flow is directed through this groove to make a "shhh!" sound.
5. Place a hand on your throat—you have to *stop* voicing here to say /ʃ/.
6. Stress your "pose" to get it right and repeat multiple times until it feels comfortable.
7. Practice each sound in the initial, medial, and final positions within words.
8. Graduate to sentences after completing the word isolation drills.

Exceptions: /ʃ/ in "-tion" and "-sion"

-tion	IPA /ʃn/	-sion	IPA /ʃn/
notion		mansion	
sanction		permission	
caution		pension	
malformation		recession	
reconstruction		progression	

Your List of Exception Words with /ʃ/ in "-tion" and "-sion"

-tion	IPA	-sion	IPA

Exceptions: /ʃ/ in "-ious" and "-ial"

-ious	IPA /ʃʌs/	-ial	IPA /ʃl/
cautious		social	
gracious		essential	
luscious		financial	
precious		national	
conscious		official	

Your List of Exception Words with /ʃ/ in "-ious" and "-ial"

-ious	IPA /ʃʌs/	-ial	IPA /ʃl/

Exceptions: /ʃ/ in "ch" and Other Words

ch-	IPA /tʃ/ as /ʃ/	Other Spellings	IPA
chef		musicians	
Chevy		dietitian	
chalet		suspicion	
charade		luxury	
chenille		tissue	

Your List of /ʃ/ in "ch" and Other Words

ch-	IPA /tʃ/ as /ʃ/	Other Spellings	IPA

Words with /ʃ/ in Initial, Medial, and Final Positions

Initial	IPA	Medial	IPA	Final	IPA
shake		dishes		clash	
shame		cushion		blush	
shared		courtship		plush	
shears		fashion		dish	
sheath		flashback		fish	

Your List of Words with /ʃ/

Initial	IPA	Medial	IPA	Final	IPA

Multisyllable Words with /ʃ/ in Initial, Medial and Final Positions

Initial	IPA	Medial	IPA	Final	IPA
Shakespeare		British Isles		anguish	
shameful		bean shooter		blemish	
shampoo		penmanship		flourish	
shamrock		pressure		catfish	
shepherd		brushing		British	

Your List of Multisyllable /ʃ/ Words

Initial	IPA	Medial	IPA	Final	IPA

/ʒ/ as in "vision"

1. Raise the tip of your tongue toward the roof of your mouth, behind the upper teeth.
2. Place the sides of the tongue in contact with the inner surfaces of the upper teeth.
3. This creates a small fold along the midline of the tongue.
4. Air flow is directed through this fold to make the /ʒ/ sound.
5. Place a hand on your throat—you have to *feel* voicing here to say /ʒ/.
6. Stress your "pose" to get it right and repeat multiple times until it feels comfortable.
7. Practice each sound in the initial, medial, and final positions within words.
8. Graduate to sentences after performing the word isolation drills.

Words with /ʒ/ in Initial, Medial, and Final Positions

Initial	IPA	Medial	IPA	Final	IPA
Jacques		confusion		rouge	
		amnesia		beige	
		casual		garage	
		decision		collage	
		division		massage	

Your List of /ʒ/ Words

Initial	IPA	Medial	IPA	Final	IPA

Sentences /ʃ/ and /ʒ/

1. Are Persian carpets expensive to buy?
2. Measure the water before you pour it in.
3. Asia is a big continent.
4. The flock of sheep is precious to the farmer.
5. She used shortening instead of butter in the cake.
6. Don't be obnoxious to the cashier.
7. Hardships are like obstacle courses that you can jump over.
8. Fill in "Caucasian female" on your application.
9. Regain your composure before you go back into the room.
10. Sam has aphasia because he experienced a stroke.
11. Hoosiers are proud of their basketball team.
12. We know a publisher that can help Josh.
13. Have you made the decision to go to grad school?
14. There was some confusion regarding the time of the party.
15. Please leave the garage open for my cousin.

16. They found the fuselage of the plane scattered everywhere.

17. What is this mish-mash we are eating?

18. Can you visualize the growth of this business venture?

19. Tina and Donna live in Baton Rouge.

20. We came by to wish you bon voyage.

Minimal Pairs /t/ and /d/

/t/ as in "tap"

The /t/ sound requires aspiration. So "tap," for example, is pronounced /thap/, where the h indicates presence of aspiration.

1. Stick out your tongue and shape it into a "point." Now point your tongue directly at whatever is in front of you, to "feel" the point.

2. *Raise* the tip of your tongue to touch or come in contact with the spot right behind your front teeth.

3. Apply some pressure as you rest the tongue tip on the ridge behind the teeth.

4. Allow the *sides* of your tongue to touch the *side teeth* to block the air flow.

5. Keep your mouth fairly open.

6. Release your tongue quickly, generating a burst of air (sounds like a small explosion).

7. Place a hand on your throat—you have to *stop* voicing here to clear say /t/.

8. Stress your "pose" to get it right and repeat multiple times until it feels comfortable.

9. Practice each sound in the initial, medial, and final positions within words.

10. Graduate to sentences after performing the word isolation drills.

Words with /t/ in Initial, Medial, and Final Positions

Initial	IPA	Medial	IPA	Final	IPA
tenth		Britain		date	
trick		British		doubt	
tide		brighter		brat	
tight		butter		eat	
trip		button		fate	

Your List of /t/ Words

Initial	IPA	Medial	IPA	Final	IPA

Multisyllable Words/Phrases with /t/ in Initial, Medial and Final Positions

Initial	IPA	Medial	IPA	Final	IPA
tightrope		clutter		complete	
time-out		fifteen		doormat	
tollbooth		detour		dropout	
toolbox		eighty-five		fresh fruit	
tour guide		flattering		houseboat	

Your List of Multisyllable /t/ Words

Initial	IPA	Medial	IPA	Final	IPA

/d/ as in "dad"

1. Stick out your *tongue* and shape it into a point. Now point your *tongue tip* directly at whatever is in front of you, to "feel" the point.

2. *Raise* the tip of your tongue to touch or come in contact with the spot right behind your front teeth. Keep your mouth fairly open.

3. Apply some pressure as you rest the tongue tip on the ridge behind the teeth.

4. Allow the *sides* of your tongue to touch the *side teeth* to block the air flow.

5. No air is released, and the sound is not aspirated.

6. Place a hand on your throat—you have to *feel* voicing here to clearly say /**d**/.

7. Stress your "pose" to get it right and repeat multiple times until it feels comfortable.

8. Practice each sound in the initial, medial, and final positions within words.

9. Graduate to sentences after completing the word isolation drills.

Words with /d/ in Initial, Medial, and Final Positions

Initial	IPA	Medial	IPA	Final	IPA
dandruff		riding		plead	
delight		roadway		paid	
demand		ridden		should	
denim		Rudolph		rode	
depot		sudden		rod	

Your List of /d/ Words

Initial	IPA	Medial	IPA	Final	IPA

*Multisyllable Words with /**d**/ in Initial, Medial and Final Positions*

Initial	IPA	Medial	IPA	Final	IPA
deposit		medial		junk food	
description		moderate		attitude	
designate		powder room		appointed	
dialogue		baby doll		brotherhood	
dimension		data disk		expected	

*Your List of Multisyllable /**d**/ Words*

Initial	IPA	Medial	IPA	Final	IPA

*Sentences with /**t**/ and /**d**/*

Identify the presence or absence of *aspiration* and *voicing* to isolate "correct" pronunciation.

1. The new restaurant is the talk of the town.
2. Tea for two, please.
3. Sears Tower in Chicago is a tall tower.
4. Tony and Tina's wedding is a terrific show.
5. Is she working in the den?
6. "Guiding Light" is a soap opera.
7. Dim the lights please.
8. I could braid your hair.
9. Pat takes care of fifty kittens.
10. Take route twenty-two into the city.
11. That teenager is trying to clean up his clutter.
12. Dan has to meet the deadline by Friday.
13. The aircraft took off at fifteen-forty hours.
14. Camping out in the wilderness was wonderful.
15. The construction of an underground subway is under way.

16. She could not decipher his Morse code.
17. Tina is a Democrat and Tom is an Independent.
18. Ten diplomats arrived at the Marriott (hotel) on Tuesday.
19. What is available for takeout from that restaurant?
20. Tim is playing in the tree house with his friends.

Minimal Pairs /θ/and /ð/

/θ/ as in "thank"

1. Place the tip of your tongue to touch the bottom edge of your upper front teeth.
2. This is to create obstruction to the air flow.
3. Release your tongue to produce the sound.
4. You should feel air escaping through your lips.
5. Place a hand on your throat—you have to *stop* voicing here to clearly say /θ/.
6. Stress your "pose" to get it right and repeat multiple times until it feels comfortable.
7. Practice each sound in the initial, medial, and final positions within words.
8. Graduate to sentences after completing the word isolation drills.

Words with /θ/ in Initial, Medial, and Final Positions

Initial	IPA	Medial	IPA	Final	IPA
third		Kathy		moth	
thirst		method		myth	
thong		mothballs		mouth	
thorn		mouthful		path	
thought		mouthpiece		Ruth	

Your List of /θ/ Words

Initial	IPA	Medial	IPA	Final	IPA

Multisyllable Words with /θ/ in Initial, Medial and Final Positions

Initial	IPA	Medial	IPA	Final	IPA
thinking cap		breath-taking		half-truth	
thirty-three		cathedral		hot bath	
thoroughbred		empathy		locksmith	
thoroughfare		ethical		phone booth	
thoroughly		faithfully		Sabbath	

Your List of Multisyllable /θ/ Words

Initial	IPA	Medial	IPA	Final	IPA

/ð/ as in "the"

The /ð/ sound is the /dh/ speech sound.

1. Place the tip of your tongue to touch the bottom edge of your upper front teeth to create obstruction to the air flow.
2. Release your tongue to produce the sound.
3. Place a hand on your throat—you have to *feel* voicing here to say /ð/.
4. Stress your "pose" to get it right and repeat multiple times until it feels comfortable.
5. Practice each sound in the initial, medial, and final positions within words.
6. Graduate to sentences after completing the word isolation drills.

Exceptions: /ð/ Words

/θd/	IPA	/rð/	IPA	/ðz/	IPA
bathed		farther		bathes	
breathed		furthermore		breathes	
clothed		seaworthy		smoothes	
writhed		Worthington		soothes	

Words with /ð/ in Initial, Medial, and Final Positions

Initial	IPA	Medial	IPA	Final	IPA
than		although		bathe	
thee		bathing		breathe	
their		breathing		clothe	
them		brother		smooth	
then		clothing		teethe	

Your List of /ð/ Words

Initial	IPA	Medial	IPA	Final	IPA

Sentences with /θ/ and /ð/

Identify the presence or absence of *aspiration* and *voicing* to isolate the "correct" pronunciation.

1. These few hours are the most precious.
2. This wreath is great.
3. Can you be here on this date?
4. They all ran to the bus stop.
5. She was calling from a phone booth.
6. Did you take a bath today?
7. This third grader is well behaved.
8. Take the meat out of the freezer to thaw.
9. This is the way to the store.
10. These people have been waiting.
11. Is she thirty-three years old?
12. Some kids are scared of thunderstorms.
13. Thanksgiving was enjoyable this year.
14. Something tells me you are withholding information.
15. He withdrew a thousand dollars today.

16. She soothed the crying baby.

17. Is the post office further down the street?

18. Her work was noteworthy.

19. She is trustworthy.

20. She won a thousand dollars.

Minimal Pairs /f/ and /v/

/f/ as in "fan"

1. Start with your upper teeth resting on your lower lip.

2. Apply some pressure as you rest the teeth on the lip.

3. Build up air pressure and release explosively.

4. Place a hand on your throat—you have to *stop* voicing here to clearly say /**f**/.

5. Stress your "pose" to get it right and repeat multiple times until it feels comfortable.

6. Practice each sound in the initial, medial, and final positions within words.

7. Graduate to sentences after completing the word isolation drills.

Exceptions: **ph** *as /f/ sound in Initial, Medial and Final Positions*

Initial	IPA	Medial	IPA	Final	IPA
pharaoh		cellophane		triumph	
Philippines		chlorophyll		telegraph	
phonics		paraphernalia		paragraph	
phenomena		calligraphy		lymph	
phlegm		hydrophobia		photograph	

Your List of Words with /ph/ as /f/

Initial	IPA	Medial	IPA	Final	IPA

Words with /f/ in Initial, Medial, and Final Positions

Initial	IPA	Medial	IPA	Final	IPA
face		afar		bluff	
feet		campfire		tiff	
fit		coffee		grief	
fowl		hyphen		puff	
fuss		joyful		whiff	

Your List of /f/ Words

Initial	IPA	Medial	IPA	Final	IPA

Multisyllable /f/ Words in Initial, Medial and Final Positions

Initial	IPA	Medial	IPA	Final	IPA
feminine		referee		plaintiff	
fashionable		signify		midriff	
formidable		infamous		dandruff	
firecrackers		referendum		fire proof	
foliage		informational		spill-proof	

Your List of Multisyllable /f/ Words

Initial	IPA	Medial	IPA	Final	IPA

*Words with /**ft**/ in Medial and Final Positions*

Medial	IPA	Final	IPA
after		craft	
fifteen		drift	
shoplifter		airlift	
rafter		graft	
lofty		shift	

*Your List of /**ft**/ Words*

Medial	IPA	Final	IPA

/v/ as in "very"

1. Start with upper teeth resting on the lower lip.
2. Apply some pressure as you rest the teeth on the lip.
3. Observe your tongue to roll backward to block the air flow.
4. Build up air pressure and release explosively.
5. Place a hand on your throat—you have to *feel* voicing here to clearly say /v/.
6. Stress your "pose" to get it right and repeat multiple times until it feels comfortable.
7. Practice each sound in the initial, medial, and final positions within words.
8. Graduate to sentences after completing the word isolation drills.

/v/ Occurring Twice within Words

English Spelling	IPA	English Spelling	IPA	English Spelling	IPA
revolve		revolving		votive	
evolve		evolving		evolvement	
survive		surviving		survivor	
valve		convulsive		bivalve	
velvet		velvety		velveteen	

/w/ and /v/ within Words/Phrases

English Spelling	IPA	English Spelling	IPA	English Spelling	IPA
Waterville		microwave		dinnerware	
swerve		radio waves		band wave	
wolves		cold wave		weave	
wolverine		shortwave		weaver	
silverware		wavelength		weaving	

Words with /v/ in Initial, Medial, and Final Positions

Initial	IPA	Medial	IPA	Final	IPA
veil		cavern		shelve	
valley		avenge		have	
vice		convey		leave	
vogue		clever		live	
voice		cover		prove	

Your List of /v/ Words

Initial	IPA	Medial	IPA	Final	IPA

Multisyllable Words with /v/ in Initial, Medial and Final Positions

Initial	IPA	Medial	IPA	Final	IPA
vineyard		diversify		deprive	
vegetate		evaporate		invasive	
vibrate		evidence		conceive	
vaporizer		invitation		decisive	
voucher		inventory		formative	

Your List of Multisyllable /v/ Words

Initial	IPA	Medial	IPA	Final	IPA

Sentences with /f/ and /v/

1. She got her first Ford Focus after her sixteenth birthday.
2. Fiona ate leftovers for dinner.
3. Are you familiar with federal tax guidelines?
4. Phillip is having an affair with Phoebe.
5. Phyllis is a traffic safety warden.
6. When does your shift end?
7. The cake turned out soft and fluffy.

8. The shoplifter was caught at the corner of Fifteenth Street and Fifth Avenue.

9. There was a theft at the loft last night.

10. He is performing at the Flagstaff Theater in Phoenixville.

11. The valve above was leaking.

12. She was tentative about her discovery.

13. His expensive venture took a nose dive.

14. Steve experienced convulsions during infancy.

15. The advertisement for the new soap was catchy.

16. The values of life evolve slowly and progressively.

17. He swerved his car to avoid hitting the Chevy van.

18. She is a survivor against the worst obstacles.

19. When are you going to move to Sunnyvale, California?

20. Everyone everywhere loves chocolate.

/w/ as in "way"

1. Start with puckering your lips.

2. Say /a/ as you open up your lips to /a/ position.

3. Your lips rest in an oval position as you finish producing the sound /wa/.

4. Place a hand on your throat—you have to *stop* voicing here to clearly say /w/.

5. Stress your "pose" to get it right and repeat multiple times until it feels comfortable.

6. Practice each sound in the initial, medial, and final positions within words.

7. Graduate to sentences after completing the word isolation drills.

Exceptions for /w/

English Spelling	IPA	English Spelling	IPA	English Spelling	IPA
once		Duane		equivocal	
someone		Dwight		qualitative	
dwarf		suite		quantitative	
square		Juanita		equivalent	
once-over		sound		inquisitive	

/kw/	IPA	/gw/	IPA	/tw/	IPA
quadruple		Guam		twice	
choir		guava		twig	
infrequent		anguish		twill	
requisition		linguistics		twinkle	
tranquilizer		language		twined	

/w/ Occurring Twice within Words/Phrases

Initial	IPA	Medial	IPA	Final	IPA
one-way		wide awake		wonderworld	
weeping willow		woodwork		swallowing	
quick-witted		waterways		well-worn	
walkway		waterworks		Worldwide Web	
Water World		workweek		workwear	

Words/Phrases with /w/ in Initial, Medial, and Final Positions

Initial	IPA	Medial	IPA	Final	IPA
witch		jaywalk		bow	
waive		freeway		sew	
wages		forwarding		tow	
waltz		reward		know-how	
weird		haywire		"holy cow"	

Your List of /w/ Words

Initial	IPA	Medial	IPA	Final	IPA

Multisyllable Words with /w/ in Initial, Medial, and Final Positions

Initial	IPA	Medial	IPA	Final	IPA
Waikiki		backwater			
wallpaper		dumbwaiter			
waterfront		castaway			
well-to-do		eyewitness			
Winnipeg		expressway			

Your List of Multisyllable /w/ Words

Initial	IPA	Medial	IPA	Final	IPA

Sentences with /w/

1. Juanita lives in Waikiki.
2. Wade is a widower from Wisconsin.
3. Edward and Owen had a reunion in West Virginia.
4. Who is willing to do the housework?
5. Someone warned Gwen about working late.
6. Waterman's children turned out to be well-mannered.
7. He felt a twinge of regret afterwards.
8. The midwinter sale on sweaters was excellent this year.
9. She ate her sandwich on the sidewalk while waiting for the bus.
10. Gwendolyn bought a twin bed and a Jaguar on the same weekend.

/ŋ/ as in "sing"

This is the /ng/ sound.

1. Lift the back of your tongue to touch the soft palate and velum (back end of the roof of the mouth).
2. This is similar to the beginning /g/ position—it prevents air flow into the oral cavity (mouth area). (Air should escape through the nasal passages.)
3. Keep your mouth slightly open.
4. Now vocalize starting with the vowel sound /i/.
5. Progress slowly to the /g/ sound and feel the back of your tongue raise to make the /ŋ/ sound.
6. Place a hand on your throat—you have to *feel* voicing here to clearly say /ŋ/.
7. Stress your "pose" to get it right and repeat multiple times until it feels comfortable.
8. Practice each sound in medial and final positions within words.
9. Graduate to sentences after completing the word isolation drills.

Word with /ŋ/ sound

English Spelling	IPA	English Spelling	IPA	English Spelling	IPA
anger		banging		bang	
angle		hanging		king	
bangle		Hong Kong		bring	
bongo		making		fling	
England		ringing		lung	

Your List of /ŋ/ Words

English Spelling	IPA	English Spelling	IPA	English Spelling	IPA

/ŋz/—/ŋ/ with plural marker

This is the /ngs/ sound.

English Spelling	IPA	English Spelling	IPA	English Spelling	IPA
bangs					
strings					
songs					
lungs					
springs					

Sentences with /ŋ/

1. Four-year-old Susan was trying to string large beads.
2. Who is bringing rice pudding to the party?
3. The box was in the shape of a rectangle.
4. He was angry after losing a Ping-Pong game against his brother.
5. Sam is flying to England tomorrow night.
6. Did you watch the marching band at the festival?
7. David had to write a report on a famous singer and songwriter.
8. What brings you to Colorado Springs?
9. Have you been to Singapore?
10. Learn the slang to completely understand American English.

/r/ as in "rat"

1. Start by saying the /a/ sound.
2. Slowly raise the tip of your tongue and curl it up toward the roof of the mouth.
3. Do not touch the roof of the mouth.
4. Place a hand on your throat to *feel* the voicing.
5. Stress your "pose" correctly and repeat multiple times.
6. Practice the sound in initial, medial, and final positions within words.
7. Graduate to sentences after completing the word isolation drills.

Exceptions for /r/

Initial	IPA	Final	IPA
wrestling		endure	
wrangle		ignore	
wriggle		sincere	
wrinkle		manicure	
wrongful		vampire	

Recurring /r/ within Words

English Spelling	IPA	English Spelling	IPA
arrears		writer	
career		uproar	
rural		revere	
horror		wraparound	
mirror		wherever	

Words with /r/ in Initial, Medial, and Final Positions

Initial	IPA	Medial	IPA	Final	IPA
rain		morning		nor	
raider		stronger		more	
rim		wrong		abhor	
roam		boring		far	
rummy		firing		spar	

Your List of /r/ Words

Initial	IPA	Medial	IPA	Final	IPA

Multisyllable /r/ Words in Initial, Medial, and Final Positions

Initial	IPA	Medial	IPA	Final	IPA
reactivate		aspiration		cavalier	
recipient		geranium		domineer	
recognition		meteorite		pioneer	
rumination		notorious		seminar	
recommend		solitary		souvenir	

Your List of Multisyllable /r/ Words

Initial	IPA	Medial	IPA	Final	IPA

Sentences with /r/

1. Her boss was domineering.
2. The school cafeteria served vegetarian food.
3. It took her half an hour to plant the geraniums.
4. The circus arena was filled with voices of children.
5. She had to wrap the gifts before the party.
6. Buy a wreath for your front door.
7. He admitted his errors.
8. What was the uproar in the neighborhood?
9. She started her career as a doctor traveling in rural areas.
10. Recurring expense has to be budgeted.

/l/ as in "lap"

1. Raise the tip of your tongue to nearly contact the ridge behind your upper teeth.

2. Be sure the sides of your tongue do *not* touch with the inner surfaces of the upper teeth.

3. Air is expelled to make the /l/ sound.

4. Place a hand on your throat—you have to *stop* voicing here to say /l/.

5. Stress your "pose" to get it right and repeat multiple times until it feels comfortable.

6. Practice each sound in the initial, medial, and final positions within words.

7. Graduate to sentences after completing the word isolation drills.

Exceptions: Final **le**, **ale**, and **ile**

English Spelling	IPA	English Spelling	IPA	English Spelling	IPA
Belle	b ɛ l	exile		casserole	
mobile		infantile		schedule	
module		juvenile		overruled	
ridicule		bookmobile		molecule	
nodule		snowmobile		miniscule	

Words with Recurrent /l/

English Spelling	IPA	English Spelling	IPA	English Spelling	IPA
fulfill		illegal		skillfully	
lapful		livelier		wholesaler	
loophole		logically		limitless	
lovelorn		lullaby		limelight	
loyalty		parallel		vestibule	

Words with /l/ in Initial, Medial, and Final Positions

Initial	IPA	Medial	IPA	Final	IPA
lapse		allure		crawl	
latch		allot		drool	
ledge		brilliant		dwell	
lunge		collide		misspell	
lucid		elated		cymbal	

Your List of /l/ Words

Initial	IPA	Medial	IPA	Final	IPA

Multisyllable Words with /l/ in Initial, Medial and Final Positions

Initial	IPA	Medial	IPA	Final	IPA
luminous		element		cathedral	
liquidate		filament		parochial	
legitimate		intellectual		perpetual	
laboratory		penalize		ceremonial	
liability		singular		withdrawal	

Your List of Multisyllable /l/ Words

Initial	IPA	Medial	IPA	Final	IPA

Vowel Contrasts Related to Final /l/

English Spelling	pill	pull	pool	peel	Pell	pale	Paul	pole
IPA								
English Spelling	till	tulle	tool	teal	tell	tale	tall	toll
IPA								
English Spelling	fill	full	fool	feel	fell	fail	fall	fowl
IPA								
English Spelling	dill	dull	dual	deal	Dell	Dale	doll	dole
IPA								
English Spelling	smile	mule	rule	steel	shell	stale	haul	hole
IPA								
English Spelling	mobile	module	poodle	puddle	spoil	inhale	small	troll
IPA								

Your List of Words with Vowel Contrasts Related to Final /l/

English Spelling								
IPA								
English Spelling								
IPA								
English Spelling								
IPA								
English Spelling								
IPA								
English Spelling								
IPA								
English Spelling								
IPA								

Sentences with /l/

1. He played the cymbal in his school band.
2. The vice-principal stressed punctuality.
3. They served shrimp cocktail at the luncheon.
4. He was belligerent about his intellectuality.
5. Is intellectual knowledge better than experiential knowledge?
6. Leah's lazy Labrador lay on the plaid rug all day long.
7. Light the lamps to celebrate the spirit of the season.
8. Speak in layman's language lest the people get bored.
9. Lucky are those who laugh, love all, and live a simple life.
10. A web of lies locks the liar in a virtual prison of dilemma.

Blends

/l/ Blends

/bl/					
Initial	**IPA**	**Medial**	**IPA**	**Final**	**IPA**
blotchy		bubbling		amble	
blameless		republic		gullible	
blaring		oblique		variable	
blunder		oblige		inevitable	
blinking		sublime		viable	

Your List of Practice Words

/bl/					
Initial	**IPA**	**Medial**	**IPA**	**Final**	**IPA**

/lb/	IPA	/ld/	IPA	/lf/	IPA
bulb		world		shelf	
Dekalb		bald		engulf	
elbow		threshold		herself	
Mulberry		withheld		gray wolf	
Albany		foretold		Rolf	

Your List of Practice Words

/lb/	IPA	/ld/	IPA	/lf/	IPA

/dl/	IPA	/ml/	IPA	/nl/	IPA
bridal		camel		functional	
candle		mammal		additional	
dwindle		formal		nutritional	
griddle		enamel		congressional	
girdle		informal		sensational	

Your List of Practice Words

/dl/	IPA	/ml/	IPA	/nl/	IPA

/fl/					
Initial	**IPA**	**Medial**	**IPA**	**Final**	**IPA**
flamboyant		conflict		muffle	
flotation		inflame		baffle	
fluency		pamphlet		sorrowful	
Fleetwood		influential		stifle	
flinching		inflexible		wishful	

Your List of Practice Words

/fl/					
Initial	**IPA**	**Medial**	**IPA**	**Final**	**IPA**

/gl/					
Initial	**IPA**	**Medial**	**IPA**	**Final**	**IPA**
gland		straggling		struggle	
glisten		everglade		boggle	
gleefully		fiberglass		snuggle	
glorious		negligence		gurgle	
glycerin		semi gloss		haggle	

Your List of Practice Words

/gl/					
Initial	**IPA**	**Medial**	**IPA**	**Final**	**IPA**

/pl/					
Initial	**IPA**	**Medial**	**IPA**	**Final**	**IPA**
plateau		applause		sample	
pleading		perplex		ripple	
plural		appliance		crumple	
plunder		employed		gospel	
plodding		amplifier		temple	

Your List of Practice Words

/pl/					
Initial	**IPA**	**Medial**	**IPA**	**Final**	**IPA**

/sl/					
Initial	**IPA**	**Medial**	**IPA**	**Final**	**IPA**
slacks		asleep		parcel	
sleet		bobsled		mussel	
slither		onslaught		vessel	
slobber		wrestling		carousel	
slumber		enslave		rehearsal	

Your List of Practice Words

/sl/					
Initial	**IPA**	**Medial**	**IPA**	**Final**	**IPA**

/spl/ Initial	**IPA**	**/ʃl/ Final**	**IPA**
splendid		impartial	
splinter		antisocial	
sphagetti		residential	
splashing		preferential	
splitting		consequential	

Your List of Practice Words

/spl/ Initial	**IPA**	**/ʃl/ Final**	**IPA**

/lk/	IPA	/lm/	IPA	/lp/	IPA
bulk		elm		alps	
talc		balm		gulp	
buttermilk		helm		pulp	
spun silk		realm		help	
hulk		palm		scalp	

Your List of Practice Words

/lk/	IPA	/lm/	IPA	/lp/	IPA

/vl/	IPA	/zl/	IPA	/lv/	IPA
marvel		chisel		delve	
swivel		damsel		absolve	
shovel		easel		dissolve	
removal		appraisal		evolve	
gravel		nasal		resolve	

Your List of Practice Words

/vl/	IPA	/zl/	IPA	/lv/	IPA

Sentences for /l/ Blends

1. They were squabbling over which blend of coffee to buy.
2. What was her blunder this time?
3. Her business flourished in spite of the fluctuating economy.
4. The director was perplexed by the lack of applause.
5. He was unemployed for twelve months
6. They bought a split-level house.
7. Do you buy groceries in bulk?
8. Use a splatter guard to avoid making a mess.
9. Where is the shovel when you really need one?
10. She acted very well as a damsel in distress in her school play.

/s/ Blends

/sc/ or /sk/					
Initial	**IPA**	**Medial**	**IPA**	**Final**	**IPA**
skewers		escape		disc	
scheme		skyscraper		flask	
skillet		sheepskin		desk	
schedule		preschool		task	
scoreboard		musketeer		frisk	

Your List of Practice Words

/sc/ or /sk/					
Initial	**IPA**	**Medial**	**IPA**	**Final**	**IPA**

/ks/ and /x/			
Final	**IPA**	**Final**	**IPA**
racks		coax	
checks		sphinx	
kicks		flex	
socks		flax	
ducks		flux	

Your List of Practice Words

/ks/ and /x/			
Final	**IPA**	**Final**	**IPA**

/sm/					
Initial	**IPA**	**Medial**	**IPA**	**Final**	**IPA**
smoke		dismount		spasm	
smear		sportsman		schism	
smart		pressman		balsam	
smudge		marksman		chasm	
smitten		dismayed			

Your List of Practice Words

/sm/					
Initial	IPA	Medial	IPA	Final	IPA

/sn/ and /ns/			
Initial	IPA	Final	IPA
snoop		science	
sneaker		fragrance	
snapshot		turbulence	
snippet		surveillance	
snuggle		audience	

Your List of Practice Words

/sn/ and /ns/			
Initial	IPA	Final	IPA

/sp/					
Initial	**IPA**	**Medial**	**IPA**	**Final**	**IPA**
sparkle		dispel		gasp	
speechless		respite		lisp	
spiked		dispute		crisp	
spoof		inspire		wasp	
sputtering		aspire		asp	

Your List of Practice Words

/sp/					
Initial	**IPA**	**Medial**	**IPA**	**Final**	**IPA**

/ps/			
Medial	**IPA**	**Final**	**IPA**
capsize		Alps	
autopsy		chaps	
gypsy		scopes	
slapstick		flips	

Your List of Practice Words

/ps/			
Medial	**IPA**	**Final**	**IPA**

/st/					
Initial	**IPA**	**Medial**	**IPA**	**Final**	**IPA**
starched		chestnut		harvest	
stemmed		chopsticks		enlist	
stirred		waistline		steadfast	
stooped		instinct		gatepost	
stubbed		hostages		must	

Your List of Practice Words

/st/					
Initial	**IPA**	**Medial**	**IPA**	**Final**	**IPA**

/st/ and /ts/					
Final	**IPA**	**Final**	**IPA**	**Final**	**IPA**
paste		chutes		admits	
haste		Nazi		duets	
waste		pizza		patriots	
baste		totes		violets	
taste		narrates			

Your List of Practice Words

/ste/ and /ts/					
Final	**IPA**	**Final**	**IPA**	**Final**	**IPA**

/sw/			
Initial	**IPA**	**Exceptions**	**IPA**
sweepstakes		suave	
swoop		suede	
swear		suite	
swindle			
swaddle			

Your List of Practice Words

/sw/			
Initial	**IPA**	**English Spelling**	**IPA**

/s/ Triple Blends

/scr/			
Initial	**IPA**	**Medial**	**IPA**
scrape		subscribe	
scrutinize		corkscrew	
screech		discreet	
scripture		escrow	
scroll		description	

Your List of Practice Words

/scr/			
Initial	**IPA**	**Medial**	**IPA**

/sks/ and /skw/			
Final	**IPA**	**Final**	**IPA**
asks		squelch	
flasks		squeak	
desks		squash	
disks		squishy	
tusks		squadron	

Your List of Practice Words

/sks/ and /skw/			
Final	**IPA**	**Final**	**IPA**

/spl/, /spr/ and /str/					
Initial	**IPA**	**Initial**	**IPA**	**Initial**	**IPA**
splices		sprawl		stroll	
splatter		spree		streaking	
splendor		sprint		structure	
spilt		spread		strenous	
splutter		sprung		strudel	

Your List of Practice Words

/spl/, /spr/ and /str/					
Initial	**IPA**	**Initial**	**IPA**	**Initial**	**IPA**

/sts/, /lts/ and /mps/					
Final	**IPA**	**Final**	**IPA**	**Final**	**IPA**
adjusts		vaults		clamps	
forecasts		felts		blimps	
tourists		consults		stomps	
requests		revolts		trumps	
druggist		quilts		stamps	

Your List of Practice Words

/sts/, /lts/ and /mps/					
Final	**IPA**	**Final**	**IPA**	**Final**	**IPA**

Sentences with /s/ Blends

1. Did you see the colorful blimps circling the stadium?
2. All her consults were scheduled by her staff.
3. The car spluttered and then came to a stop.
4. Flasks are on sale at the mall this week.
5. Reading a few pages of scriptures is a good habit.
6. She was a suave businesswoman.
7. We need permits and licenses before starting the project.
8. Todays quotes in the newspaper were funny.
9. She stirred her squash soup with a wooden spatula.
10. Tasting the spicy food made him speechless.

/h/ sound as in "hat"

1. Keep your mouth slightly open.

2. Build up air pressure and release explosively.

3. Place your hand on the throat. You will feel a slight movement when voicing is initiated in the throat area as you say /**h**/.

4. Stress your "pose" to get it right and repeat multiple times until it feels comfortable.

5. Practice the sound in the initial, medial, and final positions.

6. Graduate to sentences following the word-isolation drills.

Exceptions for /h/

English Spelling	IPA	English Spelling	IPA
who		herb	
whole		Baja	
whomever		Juan	
whose		Hugh	
why		Julio	

Words with /h/ in Initial, Medial, and Final Positions

Initial	IPA	Medial	IPA	Final	IPA
hatch		ahead		Hannah	
hinted		behold		hallelujah	
hideous		behoove		Jehovah	
hoopla		inhibit		Jeremiah	
hunted		inherent		Jonah	

Your List of /h/ Words

Initial	IPA	Medial	IPA	Final	IPA

Multisyllable Words with /h/ in Initial and Medial Positions

Initial	IPA	Medial	IPA
horticulture		incoherent	
hypotheses		behavioral	
hemisphere		inheritance	
harmonize		exhalation	
humanize		rehearsal	

Your List of Multisyllable /h/ Words

Initial	IPA	Medial	IPA

Sentences with /h/

1. Hannah plays the harmonica.
2. Harriet went to the zoo to see the hippopotamus.
3. Who wrote this humorous play?
4. He takes half-and-half with his coffee.
5. When are you going to Honolulu?
6. Heather wanted hardwood floors for her office.
7. Whole-wheat paste is a healthy alternative.
8. Inhale and exhale correctly when doing yoga.
9. Julio wanted his inheritance for his new business.
10. Heidi had her rehearsal before the holidays.

7

Accent on Accents

What kind of an accent do you have? Native speakers of American English may have an accent within their own language —for example, an East Coast or a Southern accent. People who are learning English as a second language (ESL) typically speak English with an accent that is determined by the language of their country of origin. We'll take a look at how and why this happens later in the chapter.

Every language has its own unique "sound" and rhythms. It's easy to hear the difference, for example, between the English spoken by a person born or raised in the United States and the English spoken by a native of Great Britain (or another country in which "British" English is the norm). The person who speaks American English takes a bath with a *long* /æ/, whereas the person who speaks British English takes a bath with a *short* /a/—and so on, reflecting the difference in their accents.

So we could say that *every* language is spoken with an "accent." And in fact, this is the basic definition: *Accent* is a characteristic of pronunciation that is natural in every person's speech. More commonly, however, accent is thought of as a distinctive manner of speaking a language by a *non-*native speaker. Thus, if an ESL speaker's native language is Spanish, her speech in English will be considered "accented" (because she probably is using Spanish pronunciation rules to speak English words!).

History suggests that English as a language was brought into this country by its original *settlers*—the first immigrants. Over succeeding centuries, this English has undergone many adjustments and changes, developing its own characteristics and style—the American accent. Native Americans, the original *inhabitants* of North America, had their own languages and accents that are not directly related to English. If you listen carefully, you can detect the influence of these languages on the accents of many persons of Native American heritage speaking English in certain regions of the United States.

Other immigrants whose native languages were not English also settled across North America. For example, Canada has a large French-speaking population, and French is considered one of the major languages of Canada. It is quite possible that the English spoken in Canada is influenced by French, and vice versa. And perhaps this influence also affects the accent in each of these languages.

If the influence of an ESL speaker's native language is strong, that person's speech is considered "accented." People who are native English speakers may comment, "Her accent makes her hard to understand," or "He has a heavy accent."

Dialects

Previous chapters of this book have occasionally referred to *dialect* as an aspect of language. There is no firm demarcation between dialect and language. A simplified distinction is possible, however: When two speakers cannot understand each other, some linguists consider them to be speaking two different languages. If the speakers do understand each other, they are speaking either the same language or the same dialect.

Thus, a dialect can be considered to be an offshoot of a specific language. It usually sounds similar to the language it comes from but has its own unique elements as well. These unique differences help distinguish a dialect from its mother language—the original language.

Dialect also can be defined by geographical origins and social factors such as class, religion, and ethnicity. In the United States, several dialects are spoken. For instance, African Americans historically have used a vernacular or folk-style English, and Southerners have their own variant of English with broader vowel sounds and slower speech cadence. Besides grammatical and vocabulary variations, a distinctive style of speaking—an accent—can be heard in each of these two dialects.

More formally, Webster's dictionary defines dialect as a regional variety of language spoken by a group of people that is characterized by systematic differences from other varieties in vocabulary, grammar and/or pronunciation. In a specific dialect, differences in either or both grammar and vocabulary may be noted—for example:

Grammatical difference:

He *done* it.

He *did* it.

Vocabulary difference:

This *lift* goes all the way to the thirtieth floor.

This *elevator* goes all the way to the thirtieth floor.

Similarly, numerous other word and sentence forms exist within the English dialects.

For each country, it is common for one language to be designated as the native or national language of that country. For example, the national language of United States is English. In addition, a government may authorize two more languages as major or official languages for that country if the population speaking that particular language exceeds a certain number, along with a host of other requirements. These additional languages may legally appear on official documents, or be used in oral communication for transactions of government agencies, to benefit persons who are more fluent in a language different from the national language.

For example, in addition to English, Spanish is an official major language of the United States; in Canada, French also is a major language. In India, a country that has many major languages, the national language is Hindi, and each state has its designated language, for a total of 23 official languages. In addition, English also is considered as an official language in India, as a result of 200 years of British rule. Still, each language absorbs the cultural idiosyncrasies of the region in which it is used, which leads to metamorphosis of the original dialect with birth of additional regional dialects. Moreover, each of these dialects has its distinctive manner of speech—its own accent.

Similarly when United States was established, the original settlers brought a variety of languages with them. Languages varied depending on the region—the Northeast had an influx of English, Italian, Irish, and German settlers, whereas the West Coast had Spanish and Japanese influences. Being from different places and settling in different regions these languages helped create the first dialectical variations. In addition, Native American words were introduced in some regions. Later, waves of migration brought speakers of other foreign languages into the country, resulting in the influence of various accents on spoken English.

Number of Accents

Most people speak "standard English" throughout the world. However, it is spoken in a vast range of *regional accents*. Globally, British, Irish, and Australian English speakers have their own distinguishing accents, each of which is different from the American English accent. Within each of the various regions of Great Britain, you may detect a specific accent, such as a Cockney or a Welsh accent, with regional vocabulary differences.

Within the United States you also can hear multiple accents. The New York boroughs of Brooklyn and Bronx have distinguishable accents. Other examples are the Boston accent ("Hahvahd" for Harvard); the Midwest accent, found in Ohio, Michigan, and Illinois; and the Southern accent, found in Tennessee, Georgia, and Alabama. These examples are just a few accent variations within American English.

World English

In a global marketplace of economic and political liaisons, English is the favored language for communication. Many countries have adopted English as a means of communication, especially for international meetings, business transactions, and commerce. For example, India has Hindi as its national language; however, English is used as a semiofficial language. In fact, English is the main language of books, newspapers, international business, science, technology, pop music, and advertising in India. It also is a medium of instruction in many schools and colleges in India.

Similarly, other countries also have adopted English as one of their semiofficial languages, along with their native or national languages. The reasons for this increasing popularity of English are world trade and education. Depending on where around the globe English was introduced, what is called "standard" varies. For example, English was introduced in India by the British—so standard English in that part of the world is British English.

Applied to languages, *standard* refers to what is accepted as correct in schools. For example, a standard spelling in America is *color*, but the same word in India is spelled *colour*, also used in Great Britain. In India, teachers and editors accept the second version because it represents common usage, reaching all the way back to the introduction of English by the British. However, with the influence of native language structure and rules on British English, the spoken version of this English dialect differs from the original. This is one of the main reasons why many versions of "accented English" may be heard in the business arena.

Accented English

With rare exceptions, people whose native language is not English will speak in *accented English*. It is important to remember that your pronunciation patterns in speaking English are affected by the structure and rules of your native language. For example, an Indian whose native language is Hindi will be heard speaking English with a Hindi accent. (With the number of languages in India and their differing influences on English, it probably is easier to generalize English spoken with a Hindi accent as "Indian-accented English.")

As another example, a person from Korea can be heard speaking Korean-accented English. Similarly, people in Africa, Spain, Japan, France, Italy, China, Saudi Arabia, and Mexico, each of whose native language is not English but who utilize English during business or social communications, are considered to be speaking in accented English.

Likewise, when native English speakers attempt to learn a Chinese language (China is like India in having many dialects), their speech should be considered English-accented Chinese; those learning Spanish may speak English-accented Spanish. In all of these instances, keep in mind that the speech of the second language learner is heard as accented by the *native* speaker.

Native English speakers from the United States, Great Britain, or Australia may experience similar difficulties learning other foreign languages. The most common language electives offered in schools and universities are Spanish, French, German, and Italian, although recently many Asian, European, and African languages have been added to curricula. Executives needing to learn a foreign language for business purposes utilize self-help books or audio-video tapes or may be tutored through private classes in order to fulfill their duties overseas.

Whichever method is employed to learn the new language, learning the basics in theory is very different from actually speaking the language fluently. Recall from Chapter 4 that without complete "immer-sion" in the new language, fluency in conversation is difficult to achieve. In addition, mastering the accent of another language has its own challenges. A person with an American English accent, for example, who is learning to speak Spanish will have different things to learn (or unlearn) than a person who speaks British English. A person who speaks American-accented English may need to learn the appropriate Chinese dialect and accent while living in China. The point is that the structural rules of any native language have a major influence on learning a new language in any part of the world!

Various forms of accented English—Spanish-accented English, Chinese-accented English, African-accented English, and so on—can be heard within the United States as a result of migration and the influences of the speakers' respective regional or native languages. Is one form of accented English "better" than another? That is, does a native English speaker understand one form of accented English better than another? Moreover, do speakers of one form of accented English—say, Chinese-accented English—perceive other forms of accented English—say, Spanish-accented English—better or worse than their own?

What do our ears perceive when we assign a verdict of "better" (or "worse")? Is it the "attractiveness" of the accented speech? the clarity of the accented English? Probably it is clarity or intelligibility that makes one form of accented English "better" than other forms. Speech *intelligibility* refers to the qualities of being clear and understandable. As with other properties of language, the intelligibility of the various forms of accented English depends on the influence of the speaker's native language.

No matter who the listeners are, clarity of speech in any language is vital for the message to be communicated clearly. And intelligibility makes one form of accented speech more acceptable than another to any listening audience. How do you rate your speech intelligibility, especially if you speak accented English? Notice that intelligibility is important in both accented and nonaccented (native) English or any other language. Various other factors, such as rate of speech, affect intelligibility; these factors are discussed in later chapters.

Acceptance of Accented English

Most ESL speakers are very conscious of their accents and how their speech is perceived by the American listener. Some feel that their competence is being put to the test during every encounter, leading to insecurity about their ability to deal with English language conversational situations. Foreign professionals usually are confident of their subject matter but may find oral presentations a challenge because of their accented English. Many immigrants look for acceptance both socially and professionally, so their ability to be understood within all realms of society is critical.

We all are aware that we get only one chance to make a good first impression. We know that a pleasing presentation of oneself including appropriate dress sets the stage for a good beginning. With immigrant and foreign personnel, use of the "correct" accent to make that first impression plays an important role in establishing credibility and performance reliability. Accent then becomes doubly crucial in that it can help the speaker to achieve professional distinction and be accepted as an equal.

The key is both to understand and to be understood. Isn't that what we all want, socially and professionally? When vocabulary mishaps cause misunderstandings within social or business situations, it complicates accented communication. An aware-ness of the various forms of accented English is helpful to avoid such mishaps. You may wish to confer with a speech pathologist to evaluate the intelligibility of your accented speech. In any case, some accents probably are more readily accepted than others. Still, most accents are tolerated and accepted unless speech intelligibility is severely affected and interferes with comprehension.

Accent and Speech Intelligibility

To an American, what is most noticeable about the speech of "foreigners," besides their accented English, is their difficulty in maintaining *speech intelligibility* within their respective accents. Intelligibility plays a very important part in the comprehension of any language. So long as the clarity of accented English is preserved, acceptance is easier to obtain, both socially and professionally.

Between different accented speakers, clarity of speech varies. The clarity of speech of a person speaking Spanish-accented English, for example, will differ from that of a person speaking Korean-accented English. Similar variations may be noticed in the speech of other accented English speakers that may interfere with speech intelligibility. However, none of the numerous different accented English forms currently spoken is inherently more or less intelligible than any of the others. Difficulty in understanding one form of accented English over another could be due to several factors such as the speaker's proficiency with the language, the listener's ability to detect variations in different languages, and so on.

Most ESL learners experience difficulty in understanding the American English accent as a result of various factors such as vocabulary (slang and idioms) and rate of conversational speech or speed of spoken English. They also may have difficulty understanding various "accented English" speakers from other countries, in addition to English dialects. For example, a person speaking Spanish-accented English will have no trouble understanding another speaker of Spanish-accented English but may have difficulty understanding a person speaking Chinese-accented or Indian-accented English. Different accents have different influences on speech intelligibility, making it sound worse or better to the listener.

Language and Accent Switching

"Mixing" languages is fairly common and takes many forms. Most of us second language speakers do it when we are not completely comfortable with a new language. And we all may revert to our native tongue for clarification. However, even with speakers who are fairly fluent in more than one language, the habit of mixing languages becomes acceptable in the company of others speaking similar languages. For example, among immigrants from India, both northern and southern regions, languages vary. Such persons are in the habit of mixing the vocabulary of British-accented English with their own regional language.

However, those who are fluent in more than one language also tend to practice language and accent switching. They switch between languages to accommodate a person in a group who does not know the language, or to translate. For example, in a conversation between people of different origins in an English-speaking country, it becomes a challenge to get the message across. Because everyone is attempting to improve their English, English may be the linking thread. But if one person has a language common with another in the group (Spanish for natives of Colombia and Peru), they tend to switch into words from their native language, although dialectical variations exist.

Accent switching is a little more complicated and may take years of practice to perfect. It is essential to follow the process of identifying your error sounds and all of the strategies and techniques for their correction. Having trained yourself in how to manipulate your articulators using the necessary techniques, you can "switch" between accents. This gives you the ability to switch to either of the accents—yours or American English. You can even train yourself to speak with an entirely different accent if you are feeling adventurous! That's what some actors and comedians do in order to improvise their act and add humor. So try mimicking an accent that is not yours, not American, but something different. You may surprise yourself and realize that your articulators can move differently if you train them to do so.

Most ESL speakers are very aware of their accent mishaps. Accent switching will come in handy to distract a listener away from your errors. It may even add humor into the conversation. You may feel as if you are mocking another's accent, which may make you uncomfortable. But accent switching not the same as making fun of another's accent. (After all, "imitation is a form of flattery.") If you want to speak American English fluently, vocabulary, accent, and all, classes, strategy coaching, and so forth are necessary. But certain amount of imitation is essential in your practice—you may carefully watch the way a colleague pronounces a word you've been struggling with, or you may copy your favorite news anchor's way of presenting information. Accent switching will give you confidence to *control* and *manage* your accent, to prevent situations in which you end up feeling self-conscious and humiliated. But it takes a lot of practice.

Facts and Assumptions about Languages and Accents

People assume that all languages are the same, and that with some sort of practice, they can master the new language they are learning. The key is to remember that languages may be *similar* but are not the *same*. Faulty assumptions about languages and accents may lead to delay in learning and perfecting a new language. It is always wise to approach a professional trained in the field of teaching that language to get you started on the right track.

The following list presents some facts about languages, as well as a few assumptions that may sound familiar to you:

- Most languages may have similar or essentially identical sounds. A review of all of the alphabetic/phonetic symbols in your native language and in the second language that you are planning to learn will reveal common sounds and a few sounds that may be different.

- Similar sounds may be pronounced differently, which means sounds are produced in a different place within the oral cavity and with a different manner of articulation, with definite effects on accent. For example, /p/ in English is produced with aspiration of a puff of air at the release, whereas in Hindi, a language from India, the /p/ sound has two different versions: the first, /p/, is produced *without* aspiration, and the second, /ph/, is produced *with* aspiration (the h indicates aspiration and is not pronounced).

- There may be sounds that are not present in the person's native language but are encountered only in learning a second language and hence are considered "new sounds" to acquire.

- The same or similar sounds are used in different combinations to produce new words, unlike the words in the native language. Think of a few basic words in your native language for the following English words: "hat," "pen," "milk," "cold." Compare the sounds in those words and in their English versions and observe the similarities and differences.

- Inability to make quick, sequential, and coordinated changes in the articulators to produce words with "new" or similar sounds in varied combinations affects accents. For example, the speaker rounds the lips to pronounce the English w and bites the lips to say v. To go from "water" to "vacuum" may be a challenge to a few students whose native language does not distinguish between the two sounds.

- Difficulty in coordinating and controlling the speed and direction of the tongue movements, or in maintaining consistent pressure between the articulators, affects intelligibility. For example, it takes only a slight *lack* of control to turn a /p/ (without aspiration) into /pah/ (with aspiration) or into /f/, or even /s/ into /t/. Observe the tongue position and the air flow modification for these sounds to determine how easy it is to misarticulate (mispronounce) these sounds.

- You may attempt to speak faster (increase rate of speech) under the assumption that the listener is getting impatient with your slowness in combining sounds into words, further affecting your accent and clarity of speech. Most people speak at a habituated rate; however, whether the rate is perceived as fast, slow, or normal is somewhat subjective and may be based on the level of comprehension of the listener.

Difficulty Overcoming Accents

Erasing or even modifying an accent is no easy undertaking. Although a few people have a flair for learning languages and mimicking or "picking up" accents, success in this venture is due only to sheer hard work and perseverance. Recall from Chapter 3 that learning a new language comes more easily to a child than to an adult. The following list summarizes the reasons why learning a new language is such a challenge for adults:

- Childhood is the peak time to acquire language skills, and most children pick up any language they are consistently exposed to in their early years.

- The process of language learning is *unconscious*, *effortless*, and *rapid* during childhood.

- As we get older, learning a second language becomes *conscious*, *effortful*, and *laborious*, requiring years of study and practice. Vocabulary and grammar usually are readily mastered by the diligent student, but pronunciation and spoken communication typically are frustrating because the fluency of a *native* speaker is so hard to achieve.

- Native speech and language patterns will directly affect pronunciation in a new language, and as we get older, these patterns are resistant to change.

- Spoken and written languages are influenced by social and cultural customs within the society and the country in which that society exists. Hence, learning a foreign language also means learning about the culture of that society, to be able to "fit in."

Don't be discouraged by this list of the major difficulties learning a new language. In fact, you can use the list as a tool to frame your approach to accent improvement as an informed and systematic process.

Accent Improvement or Accent Management?

Most accented English speakers are very sensitive about their accents and whether they can be understood by their American "audience." The primary goal of any accent improvement program is to promote intelligibility, to increase comprehension of the ESL speaker's speech by native language listeners. Old habits of native language patterns have to be replaced by new or different "English" patterns. In addition, learning the idiosyncrasies of the English language, such idioms and slang, and culturally appropriate etiquette will prove to be an added asset.

Throughout this book, accent improvement is presented as a *process* to decrease the effect of the ESL speaker's native language accent—Spanish, Italian, Hindi, or other—on English, and replace it by an "American" equivalent. Learning the steps required to produce each of the vowels and consonants, coupled with practice using correct models (see the worksheets at the end of Chapters 5 and 6), will give you a broad knowledge base for your accent management program; use these tools according to your need. After completion of any accent improvement course, you can measure success by noticing a decrease in the number of repetitions and clarifications needed for the listener's comprehension, increased verbal participation at meetings, and overall self-confidence.

Your spoken English may still remain "accented," although clarity is certainly enhanced. But now you can handle verbal/accent mishaps because your work so far has equipped you with various strategies and techniques to *manage* your verbal mishaps: You have developed skills to assess your error patterns, you're aware of the nature of your articulators, and you have the skills to determine the effect of your native language pattern on English and how to put to them into practice. The next few chapters will equip you with additional strategies regarding auditory discrimination, intonation, nonverbal communication, and pronunciation. All along, you also have been gathering practical knowledge of cultural nuances, etiquette, slang, and so on, and have woven them into your speech, making your spoken language more natural and attractive. This multifaceted process surely merits the name of foreign accent *management* versus mere accent improvement.

Essentials for Success in Foreign Accent Management

Many researchers and professionals have developed their own methods of foreign accent management that have set standards for other programs to follow. The following list enumerates some general essentials for success and continued improvement in such programs:

- sufficient command of the English language
- adequate vocabulary and grammar
- ability to comprehend the idiosyncrasies of the second language
- a daily environment conducive to using English to communicate, to speed up the process (reverting to native language rather than speaking English will only delay the process of decreasing the "accent")
- knowledge and understanding of speech sounds versus alphabetic spelling
- knowledge of the exact place and manner of articulation and pronunciation
- adequate practice of the "pose" for each speech sound
- carryover of the "correct" sound to words, sentences, and conversation
- awareness of the influence of word reductions (Chapter Eleven) and modifications used within conversation
- use of strategies to overcome vocabulary and accent challenges to increase speech intelligibility (e.g., techniques such as silent rehearsal, memorization using patterns or family words)
- use of paraphrasing—alternate ways of expressing messages to increase listener comprehension
- self-motivation, dedication to practice, and determination to succeed

Benefits of a Formal Program of Foreign Accent Management: Participant Quotes

People of various professions from different countries who have participated in English and/or accent improvement classes have cited many different benefits of such programs. Some representative comments follow:

- "When I done with English school, my pay as a secretary will go up many times."—Arabic secretary in training

- "My company is planning to make deals in America. I have to help, so learning English and correcting my accent will help me."—Colombian businessman

- "My company does business with the Arabic world. None of us speaks Arabic, and they do not know French. So we plan meetings in English."—French businessman

- "After learning some English I felt connected to the international world for the first time."—Ecuadorian teacher

- "I have to maintain my English to keep up with the latest progress and techniques in the medical field."—Physician in rural India

- "With Internet and global economy being the wave of the future, English is strongly becoming the preferred language to do any kind of international business. I have to improve my accent to stay in business."—Computer programmer from India

- "I understand my children better as they are going to school here in the US. They won't escape from being naughty, because I am learning English."—Chinese mother of two

- "Growing up in Africa, I did not know so many English accents exist. I have to listen carefully to understand each accent."—South African businessman

- "I have to watch people's lips sometimes to clearly understand what they are asking."—Librarian from Germany

- "Children in my art classes always correct my speech. They think I speak 'funny English.'"—Art teacher from Japan

Summary

By now you will have recognized that you are not alone in your quest to understand the whys and hows of foreign accent management. It is okay to have an accent. How you speak is part of who you are. Accent gives you an identity, a sense of belonging to the nation where you were born. But it's also okay to to adapt your speech to a different language pattern, to become more comfortable in a new culture.

Some people may think that erasing an accent is giving up part of themselves. They regard accent elimination or improvement as too harsh or too difficult. By contrast, others, who appear to be less sentimental and emotional, are more nonchalant, deciding that "this is what I have to do to get ahead in my career" or just to "fit in." Still others may merely wish to be understood without having to repeat themselves multiple times. Whatever your reasons may be, a systematic accent management program can help you achieve your goal.

By understanding the reasons underlying why the different forms of accented

English exist and with knowledge of the various techniques to overcome them, you can make your accent clearer and more attractive and may even eventually develop the skill of accent switching. Whether your goal is erasing your accent or improving your spoken English, approach your accent program as a manager ready to supervise your personal project of foreign accent management for an optimal result: a more attractive accent.

The following worksheet provides exercises in accent awareness.

WORKSHEET 7

Accent Awareness Exercises

Personal Practice

1. Listen closely to accents among friends, in your workplace, or in the neighborhood. What do you perceive when you listen to accented speech?

2. Identify and list similarities and differences in the various accents in Exercise 1.

3. Try reading the following words in different accents that you are familiar with.
   - button
   - syllable
   - develop
   - snack
   - famous
   - beginning
   - grocery store
   - apartment
   - mall
   - library

4. How many different forms of accented English do you hear at work, in school, or around your neighborhood? Can you imitate any of these forms of accented English?

5. Trying imitating and talking in another accents. This will give your oral-motor equipment a chance to feel the difference in the movements for each of the accents.

6. Listen to radio and television personalities to hear the differences in their accents. Although some of them may be native American English speakers (born and raised in the United States), you may still be able to detect the influence of an underlying foreign accent/language in their speech. The influence may come from a close relationship to foreign grandparents or other relatives or their ties to their country of origin.

7. Speak with people from other countries. Listen to their accents and observe how they speak. Invite them to discuss their difficulties or challenges with accents. Find out their coping strategies and share yours.

8. Read the following paragraphs in different accents (other than your own). (The subject matter is just my own musings—presented with no motives whatsoever.)

A Global Cultural World

The speed at which the world is changing technically and ethnically is phenomenal. While conversing with a group of Americans, you will find each one has either European (Italian, English, Irish, German), Jewish, African, Asian, Hispanic, or Native American ancestry. And more people of color— from South America, India, the Middle East, the Pacific Islands, and other places around the world—are making the United States their home.

You will see people dressed in tunics, skirts, or sandals made with ethnic patterns and designs. Ethnic restaurants are popping up on street corners. Yoga has become a household name in fitness. The phone call to fix your computer puts you in touch with a technician overseas. In a world where population is growing more diverse every day, human relations skills are just as important as computer skills—perhaps even more important.

In years to come (if you aren't already), you will be working with all kinds of people—men and women, young and old; conservative, moderate, and liberal; of various races, religions, ethnic backgrounds, and sexual orientations; and with different mental and physical abilities. There will be different problem-solving styles and ways of responding to stress. Many of these people will have conflicting ideas about social and etiquette skills. They may disagree about eye contact signals or manner of touching. Their privacy needs may be more conservative depending on their ethnic and family background. And they may not agree about certain attitudes of behavior in a work environment.

With so many confusing differences, how will we work together in the future? Better yet, how can we work together today? How can we keep cultural differences from leading us to wrong conclusions? How can we understand one another when we don't all speak the same language? It seems to me that we must join forces to globalize the human relationship skills of compassion using the technical expertise already in place.

When people are from different ethnic backgrounds, unless tolerance and acceptance are developed, frustration and misunderstandings are unavoidable. If they are not resolved, misunderstanding creates aversion and resentment. Resentment can create stereotyping—labeling and judging people without really knowing them. Stereotyping can further lead to prejudice, irrational dislike, and suspicion without reasonable justifications. These negative attitudes can make it more difficult to live peacefully in communities, attend school together, or cooperate in different work environments. Whether we are immigrants in a country or hosts of a country, learning to enjoy the similarities and to respect differences in this culturally changing world is essential.

8

Auditory Discrimination: The Art of Listening

An important skill for learners of English as a second language (ESL), and for students learning any new language, is the art of listening. To be able to change or modify your accent, you must be able to "hear" it first. You can recognize that you do not sound like a native speaker of American English—that your "overall" accent is not the same as that of your American peers. But how do you identify the exact point of breakdown—the error in the production of a specific speech sound?

To be able to pinpoint the exact error in speech sound that contributes to accented English and then to recognize the "correct" speech sound for implementation into the accent management program require the art of critical listening. As you will explore in the exercises at the end of the chapter, it is vital to hear the difference in speech sounds in two similar-sounding words, such as "cab" and "cap," with two completely different meanings

The ears are referred to as the *auditory system*. The ability to *distinctly* hear the

speech sound differences within words is termed *auditory discrimination* and is an important tool for foreign accent management. The idea is to discriminate the subtle differences in the speech sounds to improve your accent and thereby enhance the overall clarity of your speech.

Types of Auditory Functions

The ear is an organ that is able to detect a range of soft sounds and tolerate the effect of loud sounds with amazing ease. In addition, it can sort out sounds it "wants" to hear from sounds to cut out. Although we rely on our ears to hear the "correct" sounds, we perform the act of listening mostly on autopilot. Only if it is really necessary do we sometimes "cock our ears" like dogs to pay special attention. Fortunately, this act of "active listening" is a skill that can be learned and then used to great benefit in accent foreign accent management. Let's begin with a review of the types of listening.

199

Auditory Attention

The auditory system is "tuned" to receive both speech sounds (words) and non-speech sounds. Non-speech sounds are all other sounds that do not contain the phonemes. Although we hear the sequence of sounds and words, the words are never mistaken for buzzes, hisses, or any other non-speech sound. The brain evaluates the auditory signal quickly and accurately, to recognize only language units or words. This process is termed *auditory attention*.

Auditory Acuity or Auditory Discrimination

Sounds can be identified as *same* (recognition) or *different* (discrimination). Review the following examples.

- Say the following words aloud: "**b**ite" and "ca**b**." The initial and the final letters, respectively, in bite and cab are the same: **b**. However, how the /b/ sound is made differs in each word. Listen carefully: /b/ in the **initial** position, influenced by the long /i/, is a more drawn-out sound than /b/ in the **final** position, influenced by /a/, which here is short. Even though they are the *same* letter, they sound *different*.

- Now say the following words aloud: "ca**p**" and "ca**b**." Notice the difference in the final consonants: cap and cab. Another difference is that the vowel sound /a/ in "cap" is noticeably shorter than the /a/ in "cab."

The ability to identify the differences in phonemes as they change according to the sounds that precede or follow them is termed *auditory acuity* or *auditory discrimination*. This skill of auditory discrimination is critical for modification and long-term management of accents.

Auditory Assimilation or Auditory Linking

In normal speech, people produce sounds rather quickly and do not enunciate each word precisely. Some people speak faster than others. With the usual rate of speaking, however, the words occasionally run together, replacing sounds in combination or leaving sounds out entirely.

For example, in the word "handbag," the /nd/ in the medial position can sound like /m/ because of the influence of the following /b/. So although /handbag/ in conversation may sound like /hambag/, the word is still decoded as /hand/, not as /ham/. This is termed *auditory assimilation* or *auditory linking*, discussed further in later chapters.

Listening Techniques

We talk about different personalities and learning modalities. But is there such a thing as "styles" of listening? Let's address some basic definitions first. The perception of sounds such as a door slam, a cough, or water dripping is called hearing. Listening is what we do late at night when we're waiting for the next drip of that annoying leaky water faucet!

Merriam-Webster's Collegiate Dictionary defines hearing as "the sense of sound" and listening as "paying attention in order to hear." You *hear* the sound of a car honking, but you *listen* to your favorite music. After the ears sense a sound (hearing), the brain has to determine the nature of the sound heard as non-speech or speech (listening) in order to decode the message communicated. By differentiating between hearing and listening, you will enhance your auditory discrimination and listening efficiency.

You can learn the following techniques for more active participation in this process:

- active listening
- crucial listening
- reactive listening

These techniques can be practiced in social (at parties, for example) and professional interactions (meetings, conferences, and so on). The first step is to identify the strength or weakness of your listening skills. By improving your listening skills, you will enhance your ability to identify accent variations and to self-correct your own accent—and you will become a better communicator.

Styles of Listening

Let's take a closer look at the listening techniques just listed. These techniques also can be viewed as *styles* of listening.

- *Active listening* is a style of listening in which you are alert and watchful, not only paying attention to the content of the spoken words but also being aware of nonverbal communication (by gestures or indicators of mood, discussed in detail in Chapter 10) of the speaker for believability of the message.

- *Crucial listening* is a style of listening in which you are evaluating the essential, key points and vital issues by looking at the "big picture." You are summarizing in a decisive manner and leaving out the unnecessary "fluff."

- *Reactive listening* is a style of listening in which you are alert, receptive, and responsive. You indicate to the speaker that you are approachable, open, and ready with an appropriate answer to either agree or give an opinion of the situation or topic at hand.

In addition to using these three techniques, most of us unconsciously do something called *selective listening*. For example, when several people are talking at once in a crowded room, or music is being played in the background at a party, we are able to "tune in" to the speaker and ignore the others or the background noise. However, if we hear our name being spoken nearby, we readily "tune in" to that too, at the risk of ignoring the first speaker. In this process of *selective listening*, the brain chooses the auditory information selectively and focuses on what is important to the listener.

Tips for "Tuned-in" Listening

But how is listening style relevant to your foreign accent management program? Accent modification is recognized to assist second language learners to feel comfortable within the broad scope of a different language and culture. But merely "hearing" the correct accent is not sufficient to determine whether you can or cannot understand or imitate it. You must listen *carefully*, using all of the techniques you have acquired in coursework and other formal endeavors and any other strategies discovered by chance in your learning process that work for you.

Enhancing your listening skills will improve your ability to discriminate phonemes or speech sounds, which will in turn assist you in modifying your accent and enhancing the clarity of your speech. The following list provides a general guideline for where to begin; experiment with the various techniques to optimize your result.

- Practice listening actively, crucially, and reactively.

- Use one listening technique at a time in your practice, to allow for mastery and comfort.

- Alternate between the listening techniques, or use them simultaneously to increase effectiveness in listening.

- Ask questions for clarification (to get the right message).

- Use contextual clues within sentences to make an educated guess at the "right" word that you missed.

- "Listen" with all of your senses—and pick up the feelings and messages behind the words.

- Discriminate among the various nonverbal cues you receive in every face-to-face communication (you will learn more about nonverbal communication in Chapter Ten).

Benefits of "Tuned-in" Listening

It is critical to hear the difference in articulation in the two words "plum" and "plump" so that you can say them correctly. Among non-native speakers, often the pronunciation of the final consonant /p/ is exaggerated, or the sound is completely dropped. The ability to *distinctly* hear the speech sound differences in the initial, medial, and final positions within words is significant for foreign accent management.

The benefits of perfecting the skill of auditory discrimination are as follows:

- avoids miscommunication with customers and co-workers

- overcomes the barriers to good listening (external distractions and language problems)

- raises awareness for recognizing and solving common listening problems

- assists in recognition of stress, pitch, and intonation of speech (addressed in subsequent chapters)

- improves clarity of accent, thereby enhancing overall speech intelligibility

Listener Participation

How interested and responsive the listener is to your words or speech reflects your skill in communication. The reaction of your "audience" is called *listener participation*. If no one is paying attention when you are speaking, the communication interaction is adversely affected.

The idea of speech is not just to reveal your thoughts and opinions but to involve others to participate in the topic of discussion, to move people to action, to persuade them to be in agreement, and to provide practical ideas. These goals are particularly important for ESL speakers in positions of leadership and management. If your accented speech causes the listener to judge your job performance, it will most certainly affect your career path. Without listener involvement, you may lose an opportunity to influence your colleagues, along with your credibility.

As you've been perfecting your listening skills to improve auditory discrimination and accent, you probably have gained a clearer perspective on what happens when the roles are reversed, with *you* as the speaker. If your speech is strongly accented, it is logical to assume that your speech intelligibility is affected. Strong accent variations require listeners to sharpen their attention and cue in their listening; they also watch the speaker's face or lips intently to try to decipher words or speech sounds, to avoid missing any information. You know this from your own experience as an ESL learner attempting to understand and emulate the American English accent. Likewise, American or other listeners who do not speak with the same accent as yours also have to practice "tuned-in" listening techniques.

Unfortunately, this extra effort for comprehension required of the listener may lead to inattention and frustration. The speaker may in turn perceive such responses as evidence of intolerance of persons with accents that are different from the standard accent —in this case, the American accent.

Being aware of the importance of listener participation will help you self-correct your speech and give you confidence to experiment with your foreign accent management strategies more often.

Speech Reading

Speech reading sometimes is referred to as "lip reading." It can be defined as the ability of the listener to gather meaningful information by observing the speakers' oral muscular movements and facial expressions. Use of this skill typically is thought to be limited to hearing-impaired persons. In fact, however, everyone "speech-reads" at one time or another, and with a variable degree of skill.

In speech reading, the listener focuses not only on the speech—the words spoken—but also on the way in which they are spoken using the articulators. For example, to detect the difference between speech sounds formed primarily using the lips, such as /p/, /b/, and /m/, and those sounds formed primarily using the teeth, such as /t/ and /d/, and those sounds formed using the tongue, such as /l/, speech reading may

be invaluable. To help discriminate among speech sounds, the listener focuses on the speaker's use of these articulators, and also looks for contextual and situational cues to facilitate complete comprehension of the spoken message. In addition, concentrating on the speaker's facial expressions may help reveal that person's inner feelings. This type of information may be essential to the listener, to clarify the message and to avoid misunderstanding due to accented speech.

For most people, speech reading is a subtle and unconscious technique used to enhance comprehension of the spoken word. This skill is highly developed in people who are hearing-impaired. Speech reading also is very useful to persons who, on a regular basis, must interact with second language speakers who have various accents. In general, use and development of this skill are not required. But as an ESL learner, you probably recognize that *conscious* use of speech reading will enhance your communication skills both as a speaker and a listener.

Summary

The importance of good listening for foreign accent management cannot be overstated. The first step is to differentiate between hearing and active listening. This will start you on the path to improving your listening efficiency and developing your auditory discrimination skills.

The idea is to discriminate subtle differences in the speech sounds irrespective of the word position they occupy—initial, medial or final. Being able to recognize and identify the "correct" speech sounds assists you to eliminate your error speech sounds in any of the word positions. The result will be enhanced speech clarity and improved accent.

WORKSHEET 8

Auditory Discrimination Practice Exercises

Instructions:

1. Use the CD to listen to "same/different" word lists (Word Lists 1 to 3) and sentences (Sentence List 1).

2. Use a pencil to mark the speech sounds on the word list.

3. Compare the sound that you heard with the actual sound on the word list.

4. Erase and repeat multiple times till you are comfortable with sound identification and discrimination.

5. Listen for the initial, medial (vowel), or final sound and decide whether the paired sounds are the same (s) or different (d).

6. Mark your answers in the blank column in the word list.

7. Recognize and identify the differences within similar-sounding words.

8. Make a list of your own word pairs using blank Word List 4.

9. Use different listening techniques with the same message multiple times.

10. Listen to advertisements, radio shows, and the daily news using different listening techniques.

11. Pick a radio or television celebrity you have difficulty understanding and listen every day until you are familiar with the person's accent and diction.

12. Feature identification:
    - Select a feature of a speech sound (such as aspiration on /p/ or /t/ for consonants, voicing on /b/or /d/, or length of vowel sounds /I/ versus /i/).
    - Critically listen for the presence or absence of features in the speech of a familiar speaker, perhaps a friend or a family member.
    - Note how the person uses the feature in single words.
    - Notice how the person uses the same feature in conversational speech.
    - Similarly, identify presence or absence of speech sound features your own speech. Tape recording your speech can help with this task.

13. Tape recording: Record your own speech.
    - You can record your voice reading a list of words, phrases, or sentences, and even a short conversation with a family or friend.

- You may practice your word list first before recording. Or if you want to test the benefits of practice drills, record your word list before and after practice drills.
- Record sentences from the word list, or make up your own sentences.
- Then record your voice in conversation, which may be rehearsed/practiced or casual and spontaneous.
- Listen to your speech samples multiple times to identify the features you use and those you don't.

14. Evaluating progress: You can tell if you are improving by the following:
- Your listener's reactions—interest in your words and positive response to your manner of speaking
- Decrease in number of requests to repeat words or sentences
- Compliments from co-workers and friends
- Compliments from other ESL speakers ("I wish I could speak as clearly as you")

Word List 1: Same/Different

Listen to hear if the initial, medial, or final sounds are same (s) or different (d) in the following word pairs.

English Spelling	s or d	English Spelling	s or d	English Spelling	s or d
bat / pat		brain / drain		brave / grave	
ban / pan		train / rain		sale / tale	
bin / pin		pain / main		bale / bail	
Ben / pen		gain / Cain		gale / Gail	
hen / den		chain / slain		male / mail	
	s or d		**s or d**		**s or d**
ton / won		strain / grain		nail / snail	
done / ton		back / black		male / bale	
pack / back		son / sun		tale / tall	
clock / cluck		fun / none		tale / tail	
bun / pun		Jack / quack		sail / sale	
	s or d		**s or d**		**s or d**
beer / peer		pair / hair		rail / Braille	
click / lick		hack / lack		trail / train	
knack / smack		bear / bare		pill / bill	
sack / slack		rack / lack		Jill / gin	
mare / dare		hare / hair		till / sill	
	s or d		**s or d**		**s or d**
pail / bail		jail / hail		still / till	
slick / slack		click / slick		bill / bull	
mail / nail		rail / sail		pill / pull	
tail / pail		kick / click		dull / done	
sick / slick		pick / kick		mill / mull	
	s or d		**s or d**		**s or d**
link / lint		tin / tint		art / tart	
dirt / dearth		fault / malt		sort / salt	
tart / dart		birth / girth		lime / lime	
him / hymn		limp / imp		amp / lamp	
stamp / stomp		stem / hem		dent / dent	

Word List 2: Same/Different

Listen to hear if the initial, medial, or final sounds are same (s) or different (d) in the following word pairs.

English Spelling	s or d	English Spelling	s or d	English Spelling	s or d
smile / mile		tile / mile		nil / mill	
stick / slick		Rick / wick		dill / dull	
style / tile		tick / Dick		gills /gulls	
stack / stake		file / vile		kill / gill	
wile / while		air / are		lean / clean	
	s or d		s or d		s or d
take / make		rake / fake		mean / main	
cake / Jake		lake / sake		bean / mean	
wake / quake		flake / flake		teen / seen	
snake / stake		bleak / bleat		sheen / seen	
stain / slain		pale / bale		slain / plain	
	s or d		s or d		s or d
bring / ring		brink / drink		mane / mine	
lame / shame		lime / slime		rink / sink	
rang / rang		rim / grim		slink / link	
wrong / song		fare / bare		tear / tear	
read / read		beer / bear		kneel / nil	
	s or d		s or d		s or d
block / black		sock / dock		knick / Nick	
sing / sling		sing / sing		ink / pink	
sprang / twang		lock / luck		snack / snake	
flock / fluke		deer / dear		drop / drape	
peak / peak		stop / stoop		fair / fare	
	s or d		s or d		s or d
pail / pail		jail / gym		tilt / till	
lack / lack		lick / lick		bile / buy	
stink / sink		sane / sail		nine / nine	
gauge /cage		Hague / vague		lunge / lunge	
seek / cheek		lent / lend		mend / mend	

Word List 3: Same/Different

Listen to hear if the initial, medial, or final sounds are same (s) or different (d) in the following word pairs.

English Spelling	s or d	English Spelling	s or d	English Spelling	s or d
dove / shove		Dave / Dave		claim / clean	
towel / shovel		gave / pave		scream / ream	
slave / slave		wave / rave		dream / ream	
crave / cave		gave / grave		team / team	
trim / rim		Tim / tin		gleam / grim	
	s or d		**s or d**		**s or d**
beep / beak		grim / grin		seat / seed	
cap / cab		gave / gape		ride / write	
trim / trim		sane / sane		wire / fire	
cape / cave		flap / flat		take / tape	
scream / screen		beat / bead		sum / sum	
	s or d		**s or d**		**s or d**
sleet / sleet		streak / Greek		brink / blink	
sneeze / snooze		greed / greet		clap / slap	
smooth / tooth		strike / strike		crap / scrap	
smoke / stoke		grate / great		crape / creep	
smack / snack		grant / rant		scrape / scrape	
	s or d		**s or d**		**s or d**
sleep / slip		smell / smell		quill / quilt	
moth / sloth		roar / rear		snort / snort	
poke / coke		ahoy / toy		coy / toy	
knack / knack		out / owl		shallow / shadow	
squabble / Mabel		bout / trout		author / otter	
	s or d		**s or d**		**s or d**
bow / bow		redo / renew		willow / pillow	
spew / few		few / view		wallow / hollow	
holy / holy		cramp / ramp		swallow /swallow	
wrong / Ron		wing / wing		scribble / dribble	
low / blow		ring / wring		scrabble/scramble	

Word List 4: Your List of Same/Different Word Pairs

English Spelling	s *or* d	English Spelling	s *or* d	English Spelling	s *or* d

Same/Different Contrasts in Sentences

Listen to hear the differences in similar-sounding words in the following paired sentences.

1. Did she get it?
2. Did she pet it?
3. She dances.
4. He prances.
5. It was a sane thing to do.
6. He did the same thing.
7. Did you find a cab?
8. Did you find his cap?
9. Please put the seat down.
10. Please throw the seeds down.
11. He tames the wild animals.
12. He tapes the sounds of the wild.
13. Save the pictures of the trim.
14. Save the pictures of the trip.
15. What is today's rate?
16. What is today's date?
17. Did you hear that screaming?
18. Were you at the screening?
19. Are you trying?
20. Are you crying?
21. Best wishes for Dawn and Dan.
22. Here are the dishes that have to be done.
23. What is the rush?
24. What is this mush?
25. Give me a call soon.
26. Meet you at the mall soon.
27. Why are you hurrying?
28. Why are you worrying?
29. Check with your bank.
30. Check the overhead tank.
31. Lock your trunk.
32. He is drunk.
33. Did you pick up today's mail?

34. Did you order the nail kit from the catalog?

35. Which team won the tournament?

36. Which teen won the Youth championship?

37. Do you have a gig tonight?

38. Do you have to dig up your yard?

39. Bill picked her up at the hotel.

40. Pay the bill and leave the motel.

41. Train the new employees the facility policies.

42. Drain the new pump before using it.

43. Provide service with a smile.

44. Give them an inch and they will take a mile.

45. There was a ban on smoking in the offices.

46. There was a new pan on that shelf.

47. She had her hair up in a bun.

48. She had her hair done up for the party.

49. Meet Dick at the docks.

50. Deer ticks are prevalent at Valley Forge Park.

51. Sally was a dear to meet them at 9 AM.

52. Sally saw a deer during her morning jog.

53. Surprise her with a ring.

54. He was so mad that he could wring her neck.

55. Is the skating rink open today?

56. Did you hear the phone ring?

57. What did you have for a snack?

58. Is there really a snake in your yard?

59. What would you like to drink?

60. Is their company on the brink of extinction?

Your Practice Sentences

Make up your own sentence pairs using the words in Word Lists 1, 2, and 3, or from your word list.

9

Intonation:
The Music of Language

Now that you're really "tuned in" to the phonemes, you probably are very conscious of correct pronunciation as perhaps the most important aspect of your speech for listener comprehension. Even with near-perfect pronunciation and accent, however, you may find that you are still misunderstood—and that you sometimes fail to grasp the meaning of what seem like simple words and phrases in conversation.

For example, the phrase "I don't care" is used very often by Americans, both young and old. Initially, I took it literally, to mean that the speaker did not care about me or the situation at hand. Of course, when the phrase is said in the heat of anger ("I don't care what you do with your life!"), it probably means just that. Eventually, however, I figured out that it meant merely that the speaker had no preference: "Should we get Chinese or Italian food for lunch?" "I don't care."

Early in my experience learning English as a second language (ESL), I lost a lot of information by listening only for the *words* that were used. But in fact it is the speaker's *tone of voice* that conveys the true, full meaning of the message to the listener. This aspect of speech, called *intonation*, reveals the feelings, attitude, or mood of the speaker, which may be positive or negative, playful or serious, friendly or hostile, to name only a few possibilities. (So it's really true that "it's not what you say—it's how you say it!")

Every language—Chinese, Spanish, French, or any other—has its own intonation patterns that constitute an important part of the culture of which that language is a part. And use of intonation in any particular language comes naturally to a native speaker of that language.

To the ESL learner, this aspect of the new language may not seem all that important at first. But intonation is a vital part of any language, and of communication overall. It is intonation—the often subtle changes in tone of voice, as reflected in the music-related qualities of stress and pitch—that enriches the spoken word to reveal the underlying message in any communication. This chapter presents the information you need to adopt the musical notes of speech that give the English language its flair.

213

Research suggests that acquisition of near-native intonation patterns is one of the most difficult tasks in learning a second language. Yet it plays an important part in promoting the intelligibility needed for reasonable proficiency in the new language. The actual degree of proficiency achieved is dependent on factors such as similarities between the native language and the second language and the student's ability to grasp new languages as well as motivation (personal, financial) to learn a new language.

Much of the material presented in this chapter is derived from research on intonation patterns and rhythms of various languages contrasted with those in English. Findings from this interesting body of literature have been simplified into practical tips for use in day-to-day conversational practice as a part of foreign accent management.

Definition of Intonation

According to *Merriam-Webster's Collegiate Dictionary*, intonation is "a manner of utterance"—the rise and fall in pitch of the voice in speech. Think of intonation as the music or melody of language; the speaker "plays" the voice like a musical instrument to create different tones and changes in pitch within words, phrases, and sentences, to add personal meaning to the communication. Intonation can express a wide range of emotional meanings that significantly affect the interaction–for example:

- excitement and surprise
- friendliness and happiness
- sarcasm and rudeness
- boredom and annoyance
- anger and frustration
- negative or positive vibes

The characteristic of English intonation is the use of stress and variation in pitch to mark the focus point within sentences. Normally, the stress goes to the last major content word (explained later in the chapter) in the sentence, but it also can also come before that, to emphasize one of the earlier words or to denote a contrast with another phrase (as discussed more fully later in the chapter). However, the rise and fall in pitch within a sentence can vary depending on the speaker's intent or emotion (also discussed later). In the following sentences, for example, listen to the difference in pitch, reflecting meaning, as you say them aloud:

- You're going. (statement)
- You're going? (question)
- You <u>are</u> going. (command)

English has a set of intonation patterns that add predictable meaning to the utterance. The major patterns are statement, interrogative, imperative, and exclamation. These are sometimes grouped as types of sentences in grammar courses. However, these broad categories can include a variety of emotional meanings (as listed earlier) that convey the attitude of the speaker. Even without an understanding of specific words, as may be the case with ESL learners, it may still be possible to detect the overall meaning of the message from intonation.

Importance of Using Intonation

Correcting articulation of error speech sounds is one way of improving accent and thereby enhancing speech intelligibility. However, another important aspect to enhance speech intelligibility is the use of tone and change in pitch to communicate feelings and attitude. It is imperative to recognize that intonation is a necessary element that adds another dimension to your message to help convey the correct meaning. Most importantly, intonation increases listener comprehension by providing additional information that can make up for any difficulty with understanding accented English.

When intonation is used correctly within sentences, it serves to highlight certain words or syllables within words that are more important than the others. These words or phrases are spoken with added clarity in order to direct the attention of the listener to their specific content—the words and syllables are stressed. By placing the emphasis, or stress, appropriately within sentences, you can attach attitude and passion to the meaning of the message. Other syllables and words that are not as important may be shortened or spoken quickly.

English places emphasis on certain syllables or words by prolonging the utterance of these syllables or words and combining them with unstressed words (obvious in longer sentences). Therefore, English is referred to as a "stressed language." English has its own rhythms, found not only in poetry, whether sonnets or nursery rhymes, but also in other forms of repetitive speech such as counting (2, 4, 6, 8, and so on). Russian and Portuguese also are stressed languages. By contrast, in French, each syllable requires equal emphasis, so syllables are not shortened or omitted, and the same time for pronunciation is required for each word. The syllables are produced in a steady rhythm, impervious to stress differences. These languages are referred to as "syllable-timed languages."

As an example, count the number of seconds it takes to speak the following two sentences aloud:

1. The <u>gusty winds</u> roared through the little town.

For most people, the average time is 5 seconds.

2. <u>What</u> in the world made <u>Leona</u> do such an <u>amazing thing</u>?

Again, the average time is 5 seconds.

Although the first sentence is shorter than the second, both take approximately the same amount of time to be spoken. This is because the same number of essential words—five—are stressed, while words or syllables that are less important are shortened. So you can see that you don't have to worry about pronouncing each word perfectly to be understood. Instead, you should focus on speaking the stressed words clearly. This is where critical listening can play an important part in your foreign accent management. Learning what part of the utterance to shorten or discard is a very important listening strategy.

As already stated, all languages have intonation patterns. Most second language learners tend to use their native language intonation patterns in English because those are the patterns that come naturally. Listeners who are not familiar with these patterns, however, may need more time to decipher the message—which may lead to miscommunication and frustration.

Because you are residing and working in the United States, an English-speaking country, it is imperative to learn the prevailing intonation. When you use the correct intonation patterns that are standard for English speakers, you will be helping the listener focus on the most essential parts of your message. The listener then understands your message quickly and can react to you promptly and appropriately, *despite* your accented English.

Components of Intonation

The components of intonation are:

- Stress (rhythm)
- Pitch (tones)

Stress

When a word has many syllables (short segments within words), one of them is always pronounced more strongly, with noticeably greater emphasis, than the others. This is called stress. For example, the word "grocery" has three syllables: gro/ce/ry. The syllable with the strongest stress is <u>gro</u>, is the one spoken with emphasis relative to the other syllables: <u>gro</u>cery.

But how can you detect which syllable gets the stress? Careful listening will reveal that the <u>vowel</u> sound in the stressed syllable or word is longer and louder (higher volume). Some researchers also suggest that the stressed syllable is higher in pitch (Sikorski, 1988). Others (Cummins, 1998), however, advocate that "normal" stress does not necessarily have a higher pitch, although pitch may be raised for the stressed syllable to emphasize contrast (as discussed later on).

Every word in English has one main emphasized syllable. This helps to create the rhythm of the language. Emphasis is used to bring attention to the "correct" word and enhance the meaning of the message. In addition to increasing the volume and making the stressed syllable longer, variation in pitch can help show stronger emotion.

For example, let's say you pose a question to a friend: "How did you like the Broadway show?" She answers: "I <u>loved</u> it!" Her message comes across loud and clear because of the unmistakable emphasis on the word "loved." But instead your friend may say: "<u>I</u> loved it!" Notice that the shift in stress to a different word in the sentence actually changes the meaning of the sentence! (We'll explore this later in the chapter.)

Dictionaries use different systems to indicate stress within words. It is prudent to use a pronunciation dictionary, rather than a regular dictionary when you are focusing on foreign accent management. The most popular system is to put an high-set stress mark (Merriam-Webster) apostrophe (') *before* the primary stressed syllable and a low-set stress mark before the second stressed syllable in the phonetic transcription of the word. The weak stress may not be indicated at all. For example, in the phonetic transcription of the word "become," stress is indicated as /bɪˈkʌm/. If the word has only one syllable, as in /no/ or /does/, stress is not indicated. Some systems use the stress indicator *after* the stressed syllable, whereas others may underscore the stressed syllable. You may have to do some research on pronunciation systems or markers before you decide to purchase a dictionary for yourself.

Different Forms of Stress Patterns

The study of stress usually focuses on words that bring out the meaning and emotions within sentences. For the purpose of foreign accent management, however, it is essential to explore the effects of other stress patterns (syllables) on the pronunciation of short (simple) and long (compound) words.

Syllable Stress

A *syllable* is a unit of spoken language that is larger than a segment but smaller than a word and is made up of speech sounds in various combinations. When an English word has more than one syllable, one of the syllables must be stressed. The syllable that is emphasized is called the *stressed syllable*, whereas the others are *unstressed*. (We'll explore more on syllables in Chapter 11.)

In the following examples, the stressed syllables are underscored. When you say the words aloud, notice the difference in tone, length, and loudness between the stressed and the unstressed syllables.

computer	languages
pronunciation	develop

Also notice that the stress is not on the same syllable within each word. In "computer" and "develop," the stress is on the second syllable; in "languages," it is on the first syllable; and in the word "pronunciation," it is on the fourth syllable. So how do we detect the syllable that needs to be stressed?

Position of the Stress

It is important to remember that in English, the stress is not always on the same syllable of words, unlike in some languages, in which the stress is always in the same place in all word. For example, in Czech, the stress is always on the *first* syllable, in French on the *last* syllable, and in Polish on the *second to the last* syllable. In English, stress may be on the first, on the second, occasionally on the third, or even on the fourth, as we saw in the previous examples.

Although the stressed syllable in English varies in different words, *the position of the stress within each word is almost always fixed.* For example, the word "remember" has three syllables: **re/mem/ber**. The stressed syllable is mem, so the correct pronunciation, as indicated with an underscore for the stress, is re**mem**ber. In this word, the stress will *always* be on the second syllable (**mem**), *never* on the first (**re**) or the third (**ber**).

Now try saying "remember" with the stress on the first syllable—**re**member—or on the third syllable—remem**ber**. These other pronunciations are *not* acceptable in Standard English. Non-native English speakers who put the stress on the wrong syllable (**re** or **ber**) may be using the stress patterns of their native language and not that of English.

Variations in Stress Position

In the following examples, observe the position of syllable stress when you say the word out loud. The stressed syllables are underscored.

- First syllable stress words

  any

  uncle

  manage

  seldom

  mango

- Second syllable stress words

  un**til**

  be**come**

  re**main**

  zuc**chi**ni

  lin**gui**ni

- Third syllable stress words

  compre**hend**ing

  edu**ca**tion

  demo**cra**tic

  punctu**a**lity

  claustro**pho**bia

Notice that the position of stress moves from the first to the second or the third syllable as the number of syllables in the words increases.

Another feature of English is that the syllable stress changes or shifts when the form of the word changes, such as from a verb to a noun to an adjective. In the following examples, observe the stress changes based on the *form* of the word:

photo	(IPA: **foto**)
photograph	(IPA: **fotəgræf**)
pho**to**grapher	(IPA: **fətagrʌfɚ**)
pho**to**graphy	(IPA: **fətagrʌfɪ**)
pho**to**graphic	(IPA: **fətagrʌfɪk**)

Word Stress

When we read a sentence "normally" (without giving any word any specific or extra emphasis), each phrase in a sentence has one word that is automatically stressed.

This word is referred to as the *content word* in that phrase. Content words are those that carry the meaning or the feeling within the message. In general, the longer the sentence, the greater the number of content words. The <u>last</u> content word in the <u>last</u> phrase of the sentence often is the most stressed in the sentence. In the following example sentences, observe the position of the stressed word.

Example 1

The shiny car / has been parked / in the <u>gar</u>age.

Many people / often read / the business section / of the <u>news</u>paper.

The manager / called a meeting / to discuss the current issues / within the <u>com</u>pany.

The next two examples are slightly different. Say the sentence in Example 2a aloud and observe the presence of the stressed words.

Example 2a

<u>She</u> can come on <u>Tues</u>day.
(underscore = stress)

Notice that when the word "can" is used in a *positive* form, it typically is not stressed. (It actually is spoken quickly or condensed.) However, with "can't," the stress is enhanced to indicate its *negative* form, as in the following sentence:

Example 2b

<u>She can't</u> come on <u>Tues</u>day.
(underscore = stress)

Notice the additional stress in Example 2b, to support the difference in meaning.

One of the reasons for misunderstanding in speech is the incorrect placement of stress. To address this problem, a helpful beginning is to distinguish between stressed and non-stressed words using *grammatical* terminology.

All words can be classified as *content words* or *function words*. Stressed words are considered content words or lexical words. Content words can be divided into the following categories:

- nouns—*examples*: Maggie, bedroom, apple, toothbrush, Tuesday
- principal (main) verbs—*examples*: visit, come, act, construct
- adjectives—*examples*: gorgeous, motivating, creative
- adverbs—*examples*: often, carefully, cautiously

Non-stressed words are described as function words or grammatical words and also can be divided into categories:

- determiners—*examples*: the, a, some, a few
- auxiliary verbs—*examples*: am, can, don't, were
- prepositions—*examples*: in, on, before, under, next to, opposite
- conjunctions—*examples*: and, but, as, while
- pronouns—*examples*: she, us, they

In Standard English, typically the nouns carry the weight of the sentence, while the rest of the words merely support. Although verbs may carry information, they usually don't receive the crucial stress of a "first-time" noun. But in the following pair of sentences, the second sentence contains a stressed verb:

Children like **cookies**.

They **eat** them for a snack.

Notice that the information has been introduced in the first sentence. And then is repeated through the use of pronouns in the subsequent sentence, the intonation shifts to the verb.

Phrasal Stress

Phrasal stress refers to the stress on the main word in each phrase in a sentence. This may sometimes be referred to as *sentence stress* when it relates to longer sentences. Each sentence that consists of multiple phrases has a stressed word within each phrase, with the most stressed word in the last phrase. The stress on that word shows not only that the word is important but also that the sentence is ending.

In the following sentences, notice the stressed words in each phrase as you move from one phrase to the next. Exaggerate the pauses and the stresses as you say the sentences aloud, and pay attention to the message being conveyed.

> **Ma**ny people / often **read** / the **busi**ness section / of the **news**paper.

> The **ma**nager / called a **meet**ing / to discuss the current **iss**ues / within the **com**pany.

You can even experiment with emphasizing another word in one of the sentences, which will change the phrasal or sentence stress. Then observe the effect of this change on how the message is conveyed: The sentence will not sound "right," or will no longer convey the same meaning. If you want to convey a *different* meaning, however, then changing the word stress may be an acceptable way of accomplishing this:

> **I** / will **nev**er go / to the **park** / a**gain**.

> **I** / will **nev**er go / to the **park** / again.

In ESL speakers, intonation confusion occurs because of lack of knowledge of the standard rhythms of English language. By placing the stress on different or inappropriate words, the ESL speaker upsets the musical notes within the sentence, thereby changing the rhythm of the sentence. This will in turn affect the message that is conveyed to the listener. In other words, "chang-ing the rhythm" is what happens when you use the intonation of your native language in English or any other new language.

It is imperative to familiarize yourself with the conventions of intonation in English because this information can be applied to greatly enhance the clarity of your speech and your comprehension as a listener. In any case, be reassured that agonizingly precise pronunciation of every single word in a sentence is not required in order for you to be understood. Concentrate on speaking the stressed words clearly, which in turn will enhance your meaning, add emotion to your message, and thereby convey its significance clearly to the listener. As with most aspects of foreign accent management, faithful and consistent practice is essential.

For a good beginning practice session to increase awareness of English intonation patterns, try using auditory discrimination and listening techniques while paying attention to a native speaker. During this practice session, start with identification and use of syllable stress pattern during word isolation drills; this is important for accent and pronunciation practice. Then move on to identifying the stressed words within sentences, rather than giving importance to each of the syllables. We'll explore how to modify stress patterns in the section on contrastive intonation later in the chapter.

Different Ways of Predicting Stressed Words

It is not easy to identify the stressed syllables or words, especially for the ESL speaker unaware of standard intonation patterns. You may be familiar with a few survival words that you have to use daily. With some words, you can guess the pattern if they belong to the same word family (cat, bat, rat, and so on). You already know that although the stressed syllable in English varies in different words, *the position of the stress within each word is almost always fixed.*

Hence, some of the words have to be modeled by a teacher, a friend, or a colleague to provide you with an example for practice. And the rest may have to be figured out using the International Phonetic Alphabet.

Using your critical listening skills, seek out native English speakers and listen to how they concentrate on the stressed words, rather than giving importance to each syllable. Here are a few basic guidelines to get you started.

- Listen to the message multiple times.

- Listen for a longer and louder sound on the stressed or content word.

- Identify syllable stress before proceeding to phrasal stress.

- Listen to the end-of-sentence intonation and hear the strongest stress close to the end of each phrase or sentence.

- In longer sentences, the most stressed word in each phrase (the last content word) comes just before the speaker's pause between phrases (phrasal stress).

- Listen for the pauses within longer sentences that break up the messages into meaningful units.

- In *nouns*, the stress is often on the **first** syllable, as in **cen**ter, **flow**er, **ta**ble, **tea**pot, **lan**guage, **Eng**lish (exceptions on multisyllabic words like apartment, complication, triathlon, etc., where the position of the stress within words is fixed—1st, 2nd, 3rd, or 4th).

- In *verbs*, the stress is often on the **last** syllable, as in re**lease**, ar**range**, de**crease**, de**lete**, ar**rive**, re**late** (exceptions on multisyllabic words like elucidate, illustrate, envision, etc.)

- Listen for the use of emphasis that changes the focus of the message—

for example, from old information to new information: "I'd like a **small** drink, not a **LARGE** one." (In this sentence, the regular stress is indicated by an underscore, with additional emphasis denoted by use of UPPERCASE.)

- Listen for intonational evidence of emotion, to identify the speaker's attitude to the situation or topic at hand.

Stress Transcription

Let's try some targeted practice with word and syllable stress. We'll apply a technique called *stress transcription*, which can be used in addition to the preceding guidelines on how to detect stress within conversation, for maximum comprehension of intonation patterns in English.

In stress transcription, the stress pattern within words is identified and labeled to assist in deciphering the "correct" pronunciation. Stress is differentiated into many different levels; however, most commonly, *primary*, *secondary*, and *weak* or *unstressed* are the syllable designators used in stress transcription.

Let's examine the word "immigrate." Divide the word into its syllables: im/mi/grate. The syllable that has a rise in pitch to a longer and louder sound usually is identified as the primary stress syllable. The remaining two syllables are labeled weak or unstressed and secondary, respectively, in comparison.

im	**mi**	**grate**
primary stress	weak or unstressed	secondary stress

Now try transcribing the word "situation" in the same way. There are four syllables: si/tu/a/tion.

si	**tu**	**a**	**tion**
weak	secondary	primary	weak

Now say the word out loud using the appropriate stress on the correct syllable. You can see that stress transcription makes the correct pronunciation perfectly clear. Use this transcription technique to identify and differentiate stress patterns during practice (see the worksheet at the end of the chapter).

Pitch

The second component of intonation, *pitch*, is a modulation of the speech sound signal that provides perceptual distinction. We all speak words in various tones ranging from high to low, which affects voice quality. The overall intonation involves the combination of stress and pitch, creating an emotional component to convey the speaker's message to the listener.

Tones help establish a rhythm to the phrases within a sentence, which directly influences speech intelligibility and meaning. Pitch modulations in speech help both listener and speaker mark differences at the sentence level, such as in distinguishing questions from statements. For example, statements and questions are associated with falling and rising intonations, respectively.

English language also uses pitch to increase the prominence of particular words within a sentence. For example:

"I didn't say <u>fore</u>hand—I said <u>back</u>hand!"

In this sentence, the underscored syllables have a greater degree of prominence than normal, to emphasize the contrast between them. The pitch or tone variation (high in this case) is applied only to stressed syllables; hence, pitch may sometimes be confused with stress.

The tone or pitch variations may be classified as follows:

- *falling tone*—indicative of statements, "Wh" questions (who, what, why, when, and on on), exclamations
- *rising tone*—indicative of non-final statements, questions
- *level tone*—indicative of incompleteness
- *falling-rising tone*—indicative of uncertainty
- *rising-falling tone*—indicative of certainty, something very obvious

In the following examples, the different types of pitch used in each sentence are indicated.

1. It is right there.   *(rising-falling)*
2. Whatever. *(level)*
3. It is true, isn't it?   *(falling-rising)*
4. I'm not sure if he said that. *(falling-rising)*
5. What time do they arrive? *(rising)*
6. Can you get the day off?   *(rising)*
7. What took you so long?   *(falling)*
8. Are you going to be home tomorrow? *(rising)*
9. Who told you?   *(falling)*
10. Wow! That was an awesome shot! *(rising-falling; then falling)*

Contrastive Intonation

In *contrastive intonation*, a sentence is read in several different ways, with the emphasis on a different word in each version. The resulting change in meaning with emphasis of a different word is directly related to the context in which the message is originating.

In the following sets of example sentences, **boldface** type is used to show the change in emphasis on different words. (More practice sentences are included in the worksheet at the end of the chapter.)

Example 1

- I **won't** go on Thursday.
  (I refuse to go.)

- I won't go on **Thursday**.
  (I'll go another day.)

- **I** won't go on Thursday.
  (Someone else may go.)

Example 2

- I'm going to the **store**.
  (Regular stress is on the last content word of the phrase or sentence.)

- **I'm** going to the store.
  (Not you.)

- I **am** going to the store.
  (I'm not staying home.)

- I'm **going** to the store.
  (I haven't gone yet but I am now.)

- I'm going **to** the store.
  (I'm not coming from the store.)

- I'm going to **the** store.
  (A store well known to both speaker and listener.)

In addition, using the right intonation at grammatical markings helps differentiate among clauses, phrases, and sentences and among identifying statement, question, exclamation, and so on. For example, many languages make an important conversation distinction between *asking* and *telling*, as follows:

"He's here, isn't he?"
with a rising pitch verifying a question

versus

"He's here, isn't he!"
with a falling pitch affirming the exclamation mark

Intonation indicates contrast in comparing information. When you want to highlight one thing over another, you show this contrast with pitch change. Notice how the intonation indicates contrast:

- **Dan** takes **karate** lessons.
- Dan **takes** karate but doesn't **practice** it.

Intonation in Longer Sentences

When sentences get longer, with six to eight words or more, it becomes difficult for most second language learners to assign the proper stress within the words,and phrases. The prospect of persisting with appropriate stress assignment and the rise and fall in pitch, phrase by phrase, begins to seem tedious and overwhelming. However, use of stress on the key or content word that is the most important part of the message is vital to convey the right meaning.

You also may notice fellow ESL speakers trying to talk faster to complete their sentences so that the listener will not lose patience. Increasing the rate of speech, however, just makes listener comprehension more difficult—now the words run together, the intonation becomes inappropriate, stressed words cannot be recognized, and most important, the meaning is lost. Rather than directing your effort to maximizing the speed or "efficiency" of getting your message across, focus on pausing and slowing down to enhance intelligibility.

Phrasing Using Pauses

In addition to stress, there is another feature that enhances the meaning to the listener. Have you ever caught a fragment of someone's conversation in your native language, and somehow knew how to connect the information of what came before and after what you already heard? This has to do with your natural understanding of phrasing or pausing.

Pausing may be explained as stopping ever so slightly, as if to take a quick breath, in concert with use of the "correct" pitch tones, after which speech continues. Stopping or pausing after each phrase, especially in longer sentences, may help the listener ease into the flow of the topic. It's important to continue to use the correct stress within those phrases, to avoid changing the meaning of the message.

In any sentence, phrasing or pausing tells where the speaker is at that moment in the context of the message being conveyed, where he or she is going with the train of thought, and whether or not he or she is finished. Using the correct pitch at the pauses indicates to the listener when the sentence is complete. It helps with turn taking within a conversation. Longer pauses may turn into uncomfortable silences, which are addressed in Chapter 10 on nonverbal communication.

Most native English speakers speak in "chunks" and therefore need pauses to organize their thoughts. Such pauses help to organize groups of words within sentences into meaningful phrases or thought groupings. In written language, we indicate the necessary pauses by punctuation marks. In spoken language, pauses may be directly or indirectly related to punctuation marks such as commas, periods, question marks, and exclamation marks. In either case, the pauses within sentences act as punctuation marks to help create those meaningful phrases.

An effective communicator uses natural pauses and a normal rate of speech during communication. Pauses are especially helpful when the speaker wishes to enumerate more than one view or to pose a question, or to connect thoughts in two- or three-part sentences. In general, the more pauses that are used, the easier it is to understand and to hear the important elements of longer sentences. It's important, however, not to slow down so much that your speech sounds unnatural to both listener and speaker (yourself). In other words, pausing and decreasing your rate of speech, in addition to using correct intonation, will add to the clarity of your speech and make comprehension quicker and easier.

In the following examples, slashes are used to break up the sentences into phrases. In each sentence, this is the phrasing normally used in spoken English, with a pause at each slash and a slight change in intonation for each phrase.

1. The blue van / is parked / in the driveway.

2. Many people / often read / the sports section / of the newspaper / first.

3. Linda took / psychology, / writing, / and music classes.

4. We ate breakfast, / went to the zoo, / and had ice cream / for a snack.

5. Joshua got a car, / right after his sixteenth / birthday.

Practicing Intonation

So how do you put all the components of intonation together in practice? Try the approach followed in the worksheet at the end of the chapter. The worksheet activities begin with identifying with different positions of syllable stress to stress transcription, phrasing and then contrastive stress. As you use the practice sheets, you will progress from words to sentences and dialogues to conversation at your own pace. Keep in mind that success with foreign accent management relies a lot on your commitment to practice time.

Summary

An important component of your accent management program is use of appropriate intonation patterns. Because feelings are such an integral part of the human experience, they constitute a fundamental aspect of communication. The "correct" intonation patterns will greatly enhance the intelligibility of your spoken English, and your listeners will feel "connected" if they can understand you quickly instead of spending time deciphering your message.

Now you're ready to tackle the exercises in Worksheet 9–1 for practice of intonation patterns.

WORKSHEET 9

Intonation Practice Drills

Stress Identification

Instructions: Identify whether the following words have first, second, or third syllable stress.

English Spelling	**First** Syllable Stress	**Second** Syllable Stress	**Third** Syllable Stress
restoration			
eulogy			
basement			
major			
preparation			
recruit			
perform			
prepare			
because			
reside			
diet			
satisfaction			
aiming			
sacrificing			
manufacture			
sweetener			
proposal			
renovation			
celebrate			
flamingo			

Stress Transcription

Instructions: Divide the words in the following list into syllables. Then classify each syllable as having primary stress, secondary stress, or weak or no stress.

English Spelling	Primary Stress	Secondary Stress	Weak or No Stress
complication			
machinery			
dispassion			
surrounding			
disposition			
structural			
demonstration			
imagination			
visualization			
pterodactyl			
stereotypical			
agriculture			
musculature			
separating			
compatible			
disabling			
screwdriver			
cooperating			
stenographer			
accordingly			

Different Intonation Patterns Within Phrases and Sentences

Instructions: Practice different intonations with the following sentences and questions.

1. "Hi there!"
2. "Good morning."
3. "Fine, thanks. How are you?'
4. "Are we ready to begin?"
5. "Where are you from?"
6. "What do you mean by that?'
7. "Tom, may I speak with you?"
8. "Whatever you say"
9. "Damn!"
10. "Come back soon."
11. "Hey, what's all that noise about?"
12. "Once upon a time . . . "
13. "May I help you?"
14. "I'm almost done here."
15. "Maybe."
16. "She really said that?"
17. "That was a rotten thing to say."
18. "I can call back later [if you'd like]."
19. "You don't really mean that?" [do you?]
20. "What's with that attitude?"
21. "Enough!"
22. "And finally . . . "
23. "Ladies and gentlemen . . . "
24. "Do I have to do this today?"
25. "And they lived happily ever after."
26. "If you really think you can get away with this . . . " [think again]
27. "He had it coming." [it was about time— something had to be done]
28. "I am coming to get you . . . " [playfully, to a child]
29. "Don't move. I have a gun."
30. "Watch out!"
31. "Where in the world is Steve Smith? The meeting started 30 minutes ago!"
32. "I really appreciated your help."
33. "What a helpful child."

34. "Excuse me, may I have the time?"

35. "Aren't you supposed to be in line?"

36. "Show me the help and I can get the project done on time."

37. "What am I supposed to do while the document is being redrawn?"

38. "The fireworks were spectacular."

39. "The number of times I have to tell this child to clean her room—it's so annoying."

40. "I have called the office five times. All I get is their voice mail."

Contrastive Stress

Instructions: Practice contrastive stress drills with the following sentence sets. Read them aloud multiple times. You can then try contrastive stress in conversations (refer to examples on page 222).

Set 1

Now is the time for change.

Now is the _time_ for change.

Now is the time for _change_.

Set 2

I _won't_ go to the zoo on Tuesday.

_I_ won't go to the zoo on Tuesday.

I won't go to the zoo on _Tuesday_.

I won't go to the _zoo_ on Tuesday.

Set 3

Is _anyone_ using the computer?

Is anyone _using_ the computer?

Is anyone using the _computer_?

Set 4

We're having _lasagna_ for dinner?

We're having lasagna for _dinner_?

We are having lasagna for dinner.

Set 5

Someone took my parking space.

Someone took _my_ parking space.

Someone took my _parking space_.

Set 6

That sweater looks great on you.

That sweater looks *great* on you.

That sweater looks great on *you*.

Set 7

They agreed to do this project my way.

They agreed to do *this project* my way.

They agreed to do this project *my way*.

Set 8

No one wants to be taken advantage of by pushy salesman.

No one wants to be taken *advantage of* by a pushy salesman.

No one wants to be taken advantage of by a *pushy salesman*.

No one *wants* to be taken advantage of by a pushy salesman.

Set 9

Neither Sam nor George went to the game on Saturday.

Neither Sam *nor* George went to the game on Saturday.

Neither Sam nor George went to *the game* on Saturday.

Neither Sam nor George went to the game on *Saturday*.

Set 10

She walked *right* up to me at the mall.

She walked right up to *me* at the mall

She *walked* right up to me at the mall.

She walked right up to me at the *mall*.

Contrastive Stress within Structured Conversations

Scenario 1

Person A: Hi! How are you? Haven't seen you in a while.

Person B: I feel great! I got a job as store manager at the dress shop. I'm excited!

Person A: Good for you! I hope you like it. We should go out to celebrate.

Person B: Sure! I'll call you and we can set it up. I have to run now.

Person A: Okay. Catch you later.

Scenario 2

Person A:	Hi Sally! Everyone missed you at our weekly book club. Are you alright?
Person B:	Not really. I lost my job and my mom is ill.
Person A:	Oh! I'm sorry to hear that. Is there anything I can do to help?
Person B:	That's nice of you to ask. Thank you.
Person A:	I mean it. Please let me help.
Person B:	Okay, I'll remember that. I'm sorry I can't stay and chat.
Person B:	Well, hang in there. We'll be thinking about you.
Person B:	Thanks. Bye.

Scenario 3

Dad:	Todd, you are late again. We agreed that you would be home by 10 PM.
Son:	Dad, we did not agree. You decided it for me! Anyway I'm only an hour late.
Dad:	You are still late. These parties! God knows what goes on there!
Son:	You should know. Didn't you go to parties when you were my age?
Dad:	Don't talk to me like that! Show some respect!
Son:	What about my respect? You always yell and scream. I can never do anything right in your book. I'm going to my room.
Dad:	Don't walk away from me, boy! I'm not finished with you yet!

Scenario 4

Manager:	Can you come into my office, please?
Employee:	What's wrong? You look worried.
Manager:	I have some bad news for you. I'm going to come straight out and say it.
Employee:	Okay.
Manager:	The director and I discussed your recent review and decided to let you go. We'll give you two weeks to tie up loose ends.
Employee:	So, that's it? No further discussions, nothing? This is so unfair!
Manager:	Well, we have been talking about your decreased work load, inability to be a team player, and constant complaints for the past few months. The probation and plan to get you back on track have not been successful.
Employee:	Are there any other options?
Manager:	Not really. I'm sorry it has to end this way.
Employee:	Whatever! I'm out of here.

Scenario 5

Mom:	Why aren't you ready yet? Your bus will be here soon.
Daughter:	I can't figure out what to wear.
Mom:	For God's sake, you are going to school to study, not to party.
Daughter:	What do you know? There is so much pressure about looking good.
Mom:	In my day . . .
Daughter:	Oh, Mom, don't start that again.
Mom:	You have to look clean and well-groomed. Not like you're about to step on the stage for a fashion show.
Daughter:	[Sighing] All right. I'll be downstairs in five minutes. And Mom, can we talk when I get home from school?
Mom:	Sure, honey. We'll figure out something—I promise.

Phrasing/Pauses Exercise 1

Use slash marks (/) to indicate phrasing in the following sentences. Then read the sentences with the appropriate intonation according to the indicated pauses. (Refer to the examples on page 233.)

1. The red truck has been parked in the garage.
2. Many people often read the business section of the newspaper.
3. Sandra took philosophy, pottery, and advanced computer classes.
4. We ate dinner, saw a movie, and had ice cream for dessert.
5. She studied the manual, prepared her slides, and delivered an excellent presentation.
6. Would you like to start tomorrow, next week, or next month?
7. Do you want Italian, Greek, or Chinese food?
8. Are you moving to California, Connecticut, or Canada?
9. Samantha got a job, right after her graduation.
10. Toby enrolled in swimming lessons, soon after his surgery.
11. Get ready quickly, the school bus will be here soon.
12. It's starting to snow, so you better wear your boots.
13. She organized the reunion, planned the menu, and sent out the invitations.
14. Would you like to go next week, in two weeks, or next month?
15. Do you need sandals, shoes, or boots?
16. Are you buying a condo, town home, or single family home?
17. Alicia joined the YWCA, soon after she had her baby.

18. Get dressed fast, because the guests will be here soon.

19. As we get older, our memory seems to fade.

20. Since you got home early, we can go for a walk.

21. I will organize the program if it's the last thing I do!

22. After mowing the lawn, we planted rose bushes.

23. If you think you'd like to sew, why don't you buy some fabric and try it?

24. If you work hard on your paper, you will do well.

25. As you keep practicing your piano, your music will improve.

26. Why is it so difficult for you to understand the rules and stick with it?

27. I did not go to the party as my daughter was sick.

28. When you are done with your homework, I need your help with chores.

29. Should we throw a party in the auditorium or at a park, or just send them on a vacation?

30. Will you need a car or hotel reservations when you land in Chicago?

31. Will they relocate or combine the offices after the big merger?

32. You could wear short sleeves with a sweater or long sleeves without a sweater.

33. If you think that half-baked apology worked, think again.

34. Because the bank approved the mortgage, Joan and Josh bought their dream house.

35. What if you had fallen for the prank! You could have been hurt.

36. When you are a few years older, then you will understand the meaning of charity.

37. Maybe if you positioned the furniture toward the wall, you will have more light in the room.

38. Since it is too early to call it a night, let's go bowling.

39. Neither Jill, Shawna, nor Rita was able to make it to Saturday's retreat.

40. As we age, chances of taking risks or making abrupt changes decrease.

Phrasing/Pauses Exercise 2

Instructions: Practice pausing within longer sentences and paragraphs using the different reading materials you encounter every day—newspaper, magazines, and so on. Use the following passage to start your practice (the subject matter is just my own musings and is presented with no motives whatsoever). Then you may present your opinions, pros and cons, to start a discussion with a family member or a friend. This will give you an opportunity to be aware of your intonation patterns throughout the discussion.

Thriving in a Multicultural Workplace

For most of us, the way we view our work environment has changed over the past years. Besides management jargon, globalization of business has brought immigrant workers into our so-called "normal" work settings. Many people find it uncomfortable and frustrating to work in a multicultural setting. Employees get tense not wanting to change their routines and disrupt their "comfort zone." They may even wonder why all these people just don't act like regular people—like "regular Americans."

Because America is considered a "melting pot," a blend of different cultures and ethnic groups, how can a "regular" or typical American be defined? And when we assign a few selected mannerisms, attitudes, and so on to describe such an American, are we not stereotyping a group of people who may be the offspring of other immigrants (Italian, Irish, English, German) but have just been here longer than some of us?

Learning to include everyone by appreciating differences is a skill that seems essential in a multicultural workplace. It works positively for both parties—the immigrants and the hosts. Instead of taking two sides of "us" and "them" and resorting to stereotyping, wouldn't it be easier to ask questions to understand the reason for the diversity?

Hosts can focus on finding the similarities and settle on compassion; immigrants can be ambassadors for their countries and learn about the host country in order to fit in. Will this create a caring work environment for fellow employees and lead to happier and more productive days at work?

And what better way to break the ice than food and fiesta! Wherever there is food there will be a group of people converging to taste and chat. A kinship that started with an ethnic recipe may bloom to a friendship, in which people simply enjoy one another's company. That is truly global friendship.

Additional Practice

1. In telephone conversations, notice the intonation elements in callers' voices when they answer the telephone. Assign different "feelings" to the message of their words according to the intonation pattern.

2. Audio-tape yourself.
   - Record yourself saying words, phrases, sentences, and questions. Play back the tape to critically evaluate the following features: tone of voice, rate of speech, pauses, use of stress, and rhythm. Address just one feature at a time to keep the activity simple.
   - Record yourself reading a story using pauses and intonation.
   - Record yourself narrating a familiar story (fiction) or recapping an event or situation.
   - Record yourself telling a joke. Evaluate your overall delivery and the effectiveness of the "punchline."

3. To learn how to detect humor as conveyed by intonation, listen to the "masters" in action: media personalities, newscasters, talk show hosts, and so on, to observe their intonation patterns and how they use humor at the "right" juncture. For example, compare intonation patterns in the following;
   - Humorous versus serious advertisements (e.g., snack food versus asthma medicine)
   - Radio talk shows versus television shows
   - American humor and humor from your country of origin

10

Nonverbal Communication: The Mime of Language

Your foreign accent management program continues to broaden in scope, starting with the practice of oral motor exercises and moving along to incorporate articulation drills, auditory discrimination, and intonation. This chapter introduces the related topic of nonverbal communication—the numerous, often unconscious ways that people use to help convey their message without speaking.

Perhaps you have played the game of "Charades," in which others must guess the word a player enacts using only body movements and facial gestures. When it was your turn, you might have found it hard to refrain from speaking to convey the intended meaning. For this game, you and your friends would have used silly-looking gestures and engaged in absurd pantomimes, had a few laughs, shared friendly companionship, and gone your separate ways afterward. Nonverbal communication does not shut down after an evening of fun, however. It is the miming game we play all day long. The sooner we as speakers of English as a second language (ESL) become

aware of it, the sooner we can apply our understanding for better communication.

Nonverbal communication, which includes the concept of "body language," plays an important part in completing the meaning of any message. This complex aspect of language often is neglected in language instruction and frequently is misunderstood as merely a reflection of cultural differences. Nonverbal communication does have a strong cultural component, however, as we will explore later in the chapter.

The universal way to communicate is through spoken and written language, and for the hearing-impaired, sign language can be used. But there also are ways to communicate without speaking, through facial expressions and body movements.

Nonverbal communication pertains to an array of facial expressions and body movements or gestures conveying the emotional context of the spoken message and used simultaneously with speaking. As an amusing way to identify a few nonverbal communication signals, put your television on mute and watch people continuing to talk and gesticulate. You are probably familiar with many of the gestures you see or even use some of them yourself.

People in cross-cultural situations often are uncomfortable for reasons they cannot specify. Let's explore a few scenarios. For example, during a particular interaction, you may have thought, "Something seems wrong, but I am not sure what." Or on walking into a room you may have sensed uneasiness in the air. Or you may have heard someone comment: "I'm getting this vibe from him"—referring to something either positive or negative about that person's attitude. All of these scenarios involve some form of nonverbal communication.

Often the source of your discomfort within such interactions may be that the other person's gestures or nonverbal behavior patterns do not seem to fit what you would expect or be accustomed to. Unless the gestures the person uses happen to be universal, you may not understand that person's body language or expressions, especially if you are an immigrant. The result is an inattentive or distracted listener who formulates inappropriate assumptions and stereotypes regarding the other person's behavior. This is where the knowledge of nonverbal communication can prove beneficial.

For example, try "speaking" the following sentences using only gestures or body language.

- Come here.
- Stop!
- I cannot hear you.
- I don't know.

Compare the American gestures with those used in your country of origin and take note of any similarities or differences.

These examples make it clear that communication can and does take place at a nonverbal level, and that culture influences its interpretations. Research shows that there are many "channels" of nonverbal communication, including facial expression, body language, "personal space" or other spatial arrangements, hand gestures, and touch, along with intonation (discussed in the previous chapter).

Components of Nonverbal Communication

Types of nonverbal communication can be grouped into several different categories: body language including gestures, touching, facial expression, and eye contact. A few other, predominantly cultural aspects of communication, such as voice volume and the concept of personal space, also should be considerations in a foreign accent management program because they too affect the success of communication in the ESL speaker's daily professional and social activities.

Body Language

As a component of nonverbal communication, body language has been the focus of considerable research and the subject of numerous studies. Aspects of the physical presentation of self such as general appearance, personal hygiene, and punctuality are included under this topic, in addition to gestures and facial expression.

General Appearance

Foreigners everywhere in the world stand out because of hairstyles, clothing, shoes, use of cosmetics, and grooming habits. They stand out because their "fashion sense" and other aspects of appearance are different from those of the natives—in this case, Americans. No matter what their country of origin, everyone has notions about which clothing styles and other fashion accessories are attractive or unattractive, trendy or not trendy, and appropriate or inappropriate, for any given situation. Of course, these notions may change from time to time because they are subject to the effects of changes in the fashion industry.

The other behaviors of foreigners, such as body movements, gestures, use of appropriate vocabulary in specific situations, and etiquette of workplace and social settings, signal their diversity and separate them from the natives.

Body Movements

Most of us use body movements as an accompaniment to speech, to help clarify or emphasize the message. Body movements may include gestures, facial expressions, touching, and so on. People use gestures to show all kinds of (obvious) emotions, such as love, anger, or frustration. Subtler emotions, such as embarrassment, disgust, or distrust, are harder to read clearly but nevertheless are communicated as well.

Let's compare some differences in gestures between cultures with the goal of increasing awareness of and knowledge about specific attitudes and practices. In the United States, people who raise their elbows above the level of the shoulder (e.g., Italians, Hispanics) while talking, for example, may be perceived as overly emotional or even angry. Conversely, people who keep their hands and arms close to the body while talking may be regarded as stiff, too formal, "uptight," or overly polite (e.g., Chinese, Japanese). Other postures and movements such as sitting cross-legged, slouching, tapping on the table or chair arm, or excessive gesturing are considered to represent poor etiquette.

As another example, people from certain parts of India move the head in a series of circular or figure-eight motions when they are listeners. To Indians, this maneu-

ver means "I am listening—I understand," but it can be confusing to non-Indians because they are unfamiliar with the cultural meaning. On the other hand, Americans indicate agreement by nodding the head up and down or disagreement by shaking the head from side to side. These are only a few of many thousands of cultural differences identified in the study of body movements.

Standard Gestures

ESL learners usually can readily pick up a few standard gestures because they often are used by natives and are depicted on many television shows. Standard gestures that are generally acceptable within American culture include the following:

- Greetings and other hand gestures
- Summoning or beckoning
- Counting or showing numbers with fingers
- "OK" sign or "high-five"
- Head movements to signify agreement or disagreement

Greetings

Most commonly, the hands are used for greeting others and for termination of face-to-face communication. Frequently used gestures are shaking hands and waving hello or goodbye. When an argument or a fight is over, the people involved shake hands to signify a truce or peace.

Other Hand Gestures/Idioms

There are other hand movements that may appear confusing to a non-native. It is essential to familiarize yourself with these gestures in order to avoid miscommunication. In addition, you should learn certain idiomatic expressions that use the word "hand" that can be confusing to the ESL speaker.

- Waving both arms

  Waving both arms is considered emphatic gesturing and may signify "Help, I'm in trouble!" or, when performed less emphatically, may merely mean "I give up" (with a sigh after a long drawn-out discussion). So if you are parked on the side of the road because of car problems, you can wave your arms to flag someone down for help.

- Raising the hand

  This signal is acceptable to get attention in a group, to indicate that you have something to say or would like a turn to participate in the discussion. You may have noticed and picked up on this gesture if you are in a job that calls for frequent meetings.

- Giving someone a (big) hand

  Giving someone a hand means to help that person with needed assistance: "Give her a hand with those groceries." *Giving someone a big hand*, however, means enthusiastic clapping for a performer or other notable: "Let's all give a big hand to our sponsor!"

- Signaling time out

  The time out signal is made with the hands held perpendicular to each other. This gesture means "stop what you are doing and rethink." It also is commonly used in sports, when the referee indicates time out when requested by a team to address the strategy of the play. Parents or teachers also may signal a "timeout" session to stop children from fighting or arguing. With young children, a timeout is a tool for discipline in which a child who has misbehaved is made to sit in an area within the home or schoolroom that is not very inviting or distracting. The rationale is to break the cycle of misbehavior and allow time to return to good behavior or, for older children, time to understand their mistake.

- Snapping the fingers

  "It's a snap" indicates that something is easy to do. Sometimes people snap their fingers repeatedly and rapidly while trying to remember something, instead of enduring an awkward silence; in this instance, it indicates continued concentration. Sometimes people use this signal to get someone else's attention, but this usage, such as snapping the fingers to summon a waiter in a restaurant, is considered rude in the United States.

- Keeping the fingers crossed

  The phrases "I'm keeping my fingers crossed" and "please keep your fingers crossed for me" are in frequent use. The speaker also may hold up the second and third fingers crossed together. This is not really a gesture of good luck; it is simply a way to wish for oneself or others the best in whatever the venture might be.

- Thumbs up, thumbs down

  This is an age-old universal gesture that is a way to signal judgment or a decision. *Thumbs up* indicates "yes" or "good" or serves as a "go ahead" signal. *Thumbs down* indicates "no" or "bad." (You don't have to use both thumbs for these gestures, despite the name.) For example, after evaluating a new product in the supermarket, you may give your opinion, "yes" or "no," with this signal.

Another thumb gesture is used in "thumbing a ride" on a road with motor vehicle traffic (hitch-hiking). Travelers who have no mode of transportation and need a ride use this signal: The thumb is held in the thumbs-up position but is pointed in the direction of travel, typically *behind* the hitch-hiker, who walks backward while watching the road. A generous driver may stop to offer a ride (but this is not a safe way to travel).

- Shrugging the shoulders

  Shrugging your shoulders means "I don't know" or "it doesn't matter to me." In the latter case, typically it signifies that you have no preference and you are being accommodating. But it also can be used, often by teenagers, to convey utter indifference or lack of regard.

Touching

Touching is a complex and sensitive issue because preferences relating to touching differ not just by culture but also among different people and with different circumstances. So what kind of touching is acceptable? Essentially, touching can be considered appropriate in the following contexts:

- You touch when you shake hands to say hello.
- Giving someone a pat on the back is used to convey recognition or

gratitude: "You did a good job." "Thanks for your help."

- During a social gathering, hugging to greet close friends or family is socially acceptable.
- Rubbing or stroking a shoulder or an arm to show compassion or sympathy for someone in distress may be suitable in certain situations.
- People use their arms to show affection or love. Putting an arm around someone or walking arm in arm with another adult may indicate romantic feelings or family-based affection (such as between parent and child). Sometimes we put our arm around someone to make the person feel better or to show support. It also is acceptable to lend assistance to the elderly or handicapped by bending an arm for the person to use for support or offering a supporting arm around the person's shoulders.

Sometimes a few American gestures may be interpreted as offensive to people of other cultures and may lead to misunderstandings. Hands on the hips, beckoning with the index finger, and giving objects with the left hand are a few examples. To some Asian and Arabs, touching or hugging a person of the opposite sex, passing something over a person's head, and wearing revealing clothing are all considered distasteful.

Facial Expression

Facial expression ties in with emotions and feelings. Researchers state that Americans generally show more emotions on their faces compared with other nationalities. In addition, personality plays a big part in how people present themselves. We may not know the people whom we encounter, but we imagine who they are from what we see in their facial expressions and what we hear in their voices and words.

For example, smiling is a facial expression that conveys joy, optimism, and amusement and delight. It also conveys energy and enthusiasm, or confidence and promise. You smile not just with your lips but with your eyes as well. Some Asians have been known to smile or even giggle or laugh softly when they are baffled, uncomfortable, or embarrassed.

Conversely, if you don't smile or if you have tense facial muscles, your facial expression may be viewed as serious. This may be taken as an indication that the current situation is grave or that the issue under consideration is very important. It also may convey unfriendliness or lack of humor, or that you are unapproachable. These assumptions may be wrong, but the listener is going to perceive and make such decisions based on what he or she sees and hears.

Eye Contact

Eye contact is an aspect of nonverbal behavior that is especially complex and subtle but very important. Appropriate eye contact for native English speakers is to look at each other for short periods, look away, and look back again. They tend to look at the other person's eyes when they reach the end of a sentence or a point in the conversation at which they are prepared to give the other person a turn to speak.

When you listen, it is acceptable to look at the speaker's face or eyes for longer periods, but it's still important to look away from time to time. In Asia, as part of ancient tradition, respect for the teachers and elderly is shown by standing up and casting the eyes downward. More recently, although standing up to show respect may be seen occasionally, many customs have been altered to suit the ongoing changes in international business practices and the blending of global cultures.

Here are a few examples of how various types of eye contact can affect communication.

- Looking someone in the eye

  You do this if you want the speaker to believe you or to show anger—or that you are the person in control, to make people nervous. This type of eye contact could mean assertiveness or could be mistaken for aggressiveness.

- "Shifty eyes"

  Fairly rapid shifting of the gaze from side to side may indicate that the listener is being inattentive (and may possibly be untrustworthy). Inattentiveness may be perceived as rudeness.

- Giving someone the eye

  By continuing to hold a steady eye gaze, you are trying to attract a person's attention to indicate your interest. However, gazing too long and hard becomes staring, which is considered rude.

- Winking at someone

  The instantaneous maneuver in which one eye is rapidly closed and then opened is called *winking*. It is a way of saying either "I like you" or "I'm joking." Some Asian countries find winking insulting, because it may be considered a form of teasing.

- Rolling the eyes

  When you hear or see things that are unbelievable or ridiculous, or when something or someone annoys you, you may show displeasure by rolling your eyeballs upward. This maneuver indicates that although you are not engaged in contradiction, you do not accept or approve of what you just heard or saw.

- Raising the eyebrows

  This gesture indicates surprise at something not expected or not approved of. For example, if you are late for an important meeting, your boss may raise her eyebrows to signal disapproval of your tardiness.

- Making the eyes pop out/"did not bat an eye"

  When you are surprised or excited, your eyes "pop out"—meaning you open your eyes wide. For example, if a famous actress walked into your drama class, everyone's eyes might pop out. To the Chinese, however, widening the eyes often is a sign of anger.

  Conversely, some people may not show any emotion of astonishment or shock or any reaction at all. When this happens, we say that they "did not bat an eye" ("bat" here refers to "blink"). Their emotional demeanor stayed the same even though the situation changed.

In the following examples, you will notice that the situation called for the use of gestures or nonverbal communication, rather than speech.

Scenario 1

In a restaurant, you want more coffee. It's the lunch hour crowd, and you're having a hard time catching the waitress's eye. When she finally sees you across the room, you lift your empty cup. She nods and then uses her hand and wrist to mimic pouring cream, raising her eyebrows to signify

a question. You shake your head from side to side, and she nods, indicating "okay." Without verbal communication, you have managed to communicate clearly to the waitress to bring you more coffee without cream.

Scenario 2

You are with a friend at a bar. The conversation turns personal and your friend requests you not to say anything to others. You respond by holding your thumb and one or two fingers at the level of your lips, giving your wrist a right-handed turn, and pretending to throw something over your shoulder. Without using verbal communication you have just clearly indicated that you "locked" your lips and threw away the key—meaning that the secret is safe with you. (Notice that use of a *non*verbal response supports the discretion promised by your gestures!)

Isn't it amazing what nonverbal communication can accomplish? Again, television can be a good place to observe various modes of eye contact and other standard gestures as different scenarios are played out. Children's cartoons and "sitcoms" (situation comedies) are famous for exaggeration of facial expression and other aspects of nonverbal communication; such programs provide the ESL learner with a wealth of material for study. It's important to view the program using the mute button, however; otherwise, you may be distracted by the voices.

Volume of Voice and Other Speech-Related Issues

It is important to be aware how you use your voice to communicate, because your voice is a primary tool to convey your message. You should vary the tone of your voice to express emotion within any message. As discussed in Chapter 9, on intonation, pitch or tone of voice is a component of speech that conveys emotion.

When you don't produce any variation in your tone, your voice will be perceived as a *monotone*. Whether heard in a one-on-one conversation or a group interaction, a monotone voice does not produce listener involvement. It is up to you to choose to vary the tone of your voice to create interest in the listener. Being enthusiastic about speaking your message will enhance the quality of the message conveyed.

In some cultures, however, the overall pitch or tone of voice for a specific language may be higher than that for other languages. If you hear two Chinese people conversing, you will hear a pitch higher than what is standard for English. In addition, you will hear an interesting "sing-song" intonation that is natural for Chinese. Some of the languages and dialects found in India and Africa also use a slightly higher pitch and sing-song intonation pattern.

Varying your tone of voice so that your speech doesn't sound monotone does not mean raising your voice to an abnormally high pitch or volume. For example, people tend to speak louder when they are around hearing-impaired persons. However, if a foreigner takes longer to comprehend and respond to a native speaker of English, there is a tendency for that speaker to raise the voice in an attempt to clarify the information. (Much to my embarrassment, I had such an encounter during my first week in this country, when my comprehension was sluggish as a result of jet lag and all the newness surrounding me.) Most foreigners do *not* have difficulty hearing, however, and in fact raising the voice may signal rudeness and sound confrontational. Instead, a pause in the conversation may provide the time a foreign speaker needs to gather his or her thoughts to respond.

Pausing to give someone time to comprehend produces a lull in the conversation, with resultant silence. And silence for longer than a certain period of time can become uncomfortable. Americans tend to be restless and uneasy with lapses in conversation or periods of silence, unless in the company of good friends or family. If the period of silence lasts around 10 to 15 seconds, most Americans prefer to make any comment just to break the silence. But as a non-native speaker you can explain to them the need for this pause or processing time. Sometimes it will be up to you to modify the situation for the best possible outcome.

Another voice-related issue is the use of hems, haws, sighs, gasps, coughs, and throat clearing *by foreigners* to buy time in a conversation. For example, an informal study of several Spanish-speaking students from Columbia, Peru, or Puerto Rico showed that they use the sound "ay" as a fill-in while trying to find the correct vocabulary words within conversation. Sometimes they repeated "ay" multiple times: If the sentence consisted of 10 words, 5 of them were "ay." Use of such time-buying vocalizations may be considered rude and is frustrating to the listener. Bringing awareness to your voice mannerisms helps eliminate inappropriate vocalizations and will make your speech more presentable and acceptable.

Attention to Punctuality

Punctuality, agenda, and timetables are very important in the business world. Employees are expected to arrive on time, especially for scheduled meetings, interviews, conferences, and seminars. The meetings and seminars have to start and finish "right on time." The areas listed on the meeting agenda are addressed in the allotted time. Any delay in start-up or "getting behind" on the agenda tends to be considered an example of poor management practices.

However, at social gatherings the rule regarding punctuality is somewhat lax. Although the host expects you on time, it is permissible to show up a few minutes "fashionably late." Any later indicates lack of courtesy, unless this has been discussed in advance with the host or if there is an emergency.

Space and Distance

What is your awareness regarding personal space and distance? Two people conversing at the office water cooler or standing in line at the post office will tend to keep a certain amount of space between them. As a species, humans are territorial. Unless someone violates our personal space, however, we seem to be oblivious to it. Nevertheless, there is territory at the office (we have our own cubicles), in the home (guests are allowed in specific rooms only), and in public places (we mark our spot on the beach with a blanket or big colorful towel). Space applies to conversation too.

It is thought that culture strongly influences this behavior. In the English-speaking community, there is an unwritten rule regarding normal conversational distance: The speaker and the listener should be standing or sitting a certain distance apart, not too close together and not too far apart. In countries such as China, India, and Africa, the rules regarding spatial distance during conversation are fairly lenient, sometimes ignoring occasional body contact. People from such cultures are fairly relaxed in crowded settings, without a tendency to "hold themselves in."

Edward Hall, in his book *The Hidden Dimension*, talks about "standing distances" between people: "we are often unaware that distances between people in the American society are significant." He suggests that Americans create "an intimate or personal zone" in which people talk while standing approximately 18 inches apart. If a person moves closer, invading this private area, the other tends to move away. In the subway or a crowed elevator, Americans will hold themselves in to avoid bodily contact with strangers.

Altering the distance between two people can convey a desire for intimacy, may declare a lack of interest, or may be used to increase or decrease control, such as in police interrogation techniques. The rationale for this authority-based technique is that invasion of personal space with no chance for defense gives the interrogating officer a psychological benefit. In a social situation, however, unless a friend or acquaintance becomes an aggressor, the prohibition against encroachment on personal space may be temporarily set aside. Moving closer to convey a desire for intimacy may be translated as a wish to establish friendship or courtship.

In other cultures, the boundaries defining an "intimate zone" may be either closer or farther apart or may not exist at all. For example, in a conversation between an American and a Greek, Indian, or Arab, you are likely to notice the American trying to back away because the other person is getting "too close." By contrast, you may notice the American trying to get closer to a Japanese speaker, because in Japanese culture it is customary to stand a little too far away by American standards. In both cases, the speaker and the listener are becoming uncomfortable and are likely to make incorrect assumptions about each other. This may lead to stereotyping, so that the outcome of the interaction becomes tainted. A knowledge of customary boundaries is thus always helpful in promoting effective cross-cultural communication.

Personal Hygiene

How does personal hygiene relate to nonverbal communication? Because the topic of body language was introduced earlier in the chapter, all things pertaining to the body and its perception to the listener may be considered relevant. Without a doubt this is a very delicate and embarrassing issue to talk about and requires tact.

Other terms used in conjunction with personal hygiene are grooming and cleanliness. American television commercials make it very clear what are considered "perfect" personal hygiene habits. The market is flooded with multiple products such as deodorants, talcum powder, perfumes, soaps, and so on, for all aspects of personal hygiene. The message comes across loud and clear: For any interaction between two or more people, good personal hygiene is a requirement in both professional and social environments.

Of course, there is no written rule that anyone visiting the United States *has* to follow these customs. However, it is polite and respectful to adopt the general practices that prevail in any country to create a good impression, both professionally and socially. It's a good idea to be alert to such practices, and to be proactive in seeking ways to manage these issues, so that your interactions will be constructive, positive experiences.

Not all natives have excellent personal hygiene habits, of course, nor do all foreigners have poor personal habits. But standards for personal hygiene and cleanliness are recognized to vary both culturally and from person to person. Consider consulting close friends or family members to identify areas in which adaptations may be needed.

Some common signs of poor personal hygiene that can adversely affect intercultural interactions are the following:

- too much cologne or perfume
- dirty nails
- dandruff, unmanaged hair (head, ears, nose)
- talking with food in the mouth
- body odor
- foot odor
- mouth odor (halitosis, also called bad breath)

Certain foods such as garlic, raw onions, broccoli, cabbage, brussel sprouts, spices, and alcohol cause body and mouth odor. The clothing of a person walking out of a pizza parlor or an Indian, Chinese, or other "ethnic" restaurant may have a characteristic odor. Such odors, however, are not desirable at work, in class, or at a meeting. Again, these issues are not restricted to foreigners only—they apply to natives as well.

There also are medical conditions such as esophagitis or sinusitis, and certain drugs that may cause bad breath. *Awareness* is the key, followed by appropriate management including good dental hygiene and other personal hygiene practices. Alternatively, if the issue is more complex, medical consultation may be indicated. Use of products such as mouthwash and deodorants, using table napkins periodically throughout the meal, and hand washing after using the restroom usually are adequate to alleviate many of these issues.

Surviving Cultural Differences

Whether you are a relative newcomer or have lived in the United States for some years, it's important to learn to adapt to the prevailing modes of nonverbal communication in your professional and social relationships. It will benefit your adjustment to the new culture—and enhance your appreciation of your own—to work hard at developing and maintaining sensitivity and respect for all cultural differences everywhere in the world. That is the key lesson presented in this chapter: adapt without judgment.

One of the ways to adapt and survive cultural differences is by *managing* your nonverbal communication. Creating awareness of the nonverbal aspects of interpersonal communication is absolutely necessary to survive in any new country and crucial to get along in another culture. Here are some ideas to sharpen your skills of nonverbal communication.

- Identify your own habits and gestures. It is important to recognize your differences and/or peculiarities before deciding to change them.

- Be aware of your preconceived notions, attitudes, and knowledge about the United States that strongly influence the type of encounters you have.

- Ask questions to clarify what you observe, to dispel those preconceived notions, stereotypes, or misinformation on your part. Most natives respond amicably; however, you may run into a few rude people. Overlook such minor setbacks and keep prodding—no question is "stupid" or too basic.

- Find out how you look to others during a presentation or when you are nervous.

- Pick one or two essentials to work on from the different aspects of nonverbal communication outlined in this chapter (e.g., body language and gestures). Identify your practice goals within a specific time frame—for example, "Over the next 3 weeks, I will observe my body language when I'm talking with my boss."

- When you are comfortable using these essentials, choose others that are important to *you*. Ongoing practice will effect change in your communication style.

- Be open to correction by friends and perhaps even strangers without feeling embarrassed, because this is the best way to learn.

- Always retain a "natural" tone to your communication. Otherwise, you may sound insincere (or perhaps you may be perceived as somewhat peculiar).

- Find a place with lots of people, such as a shopping mall, to observe people's interaction, eye contact, gestures, and so on. Much can be learned from simple observation.

- Observe the "masters" in action—television talk-show hosts and others in the public eye. Notice how they continually involve their listeners and guests and how they move around, and their use of facial expressions and gestures.

- Be a *teacher* and an *ambassador* of your country to all Americans. The answers to some questions from Americans may seem obvious to you; however, such questions may be based on preconceived notions and stereotypical ideas, or on misinformation. In any case, you will need to develop patience for your role as educator, utilizing your English language skills.

Summary

The topic of nonverbal communication is complex and sometimes delicate. Accordingly, people tend to ignore the relevant issues, which may then become a source of misunderstanding. Unaware of the underlying etiquette, people may make assumptions leading to miscommunication. To add to the basics presented in this chapter, you can increase your knowledge base by referring to a few books mentioned in the suggested reading section at the end of the book.

Understanding body language and how it ties in with communication can assist the second language learner to overcome any feelings of superiority or inferiority and to avoid stereotyping or labeling. This knowledge also will help to eliminate mistaken interpretations and promote understanding of cultural differences.

Applying your new awareness of the various aspects of nonverbal communication will help you refine your overall communi-

cation techniques. As recommended earlier, selecting one or two aspects to work on (from the list under "Surviving Cultural Differences") is a good place to start. In addition, by playing the role of teacher or ambassador of your country of origin, you can make a real contribution, calming fears of "otherness" and opening doors to a completely new world of cultural communication.

Worksheet 10–1 presents an array of suggested activities to enhance awareness of personal and cultural differences and similarities in nonverbal communication modes.

WORKSHEET 10

Nonverbal Communication Awareness Activities

Practice and Observations

1. Handshakes
   - Are there different kinds of handshakes?
   - Try them with your colleagues to determine if a handshake can tell you something about a person.

2. Coping with stressful situations
   - Do you smile nervously or become "stone-faced" under pressure?
   - Do you yell and leave the room?
   - Do you have a nervous giggle to cover up your embarrassment?

3. Irritation
   - Do you communicate impatience by tapping your foot?
   - Do you drum your fingers or a pen on the table when you are listening to a speaker who bores or annoys you?
   - What is your reaction to the listener who is inattentive or does drumming or foot-tapping while you are the speaker?

4. Eye contact and facial expression
   - Do you know <u>where</u> you look when you are talking with or listening to another person?
   - Does your facial expression convey seriousness or friendliness?
   - Observe your family, friends, and colleagues to see if you can read their facial expressions.
   - What is the eye contact rule in your country of origin?

5. Dress code
   - What is a dress code?
   - Do you have a dress code for different occasions in your country?
   - Discuss casual versus business fashions with Americans.
   - What are the business practices, fashions, and etiquette in your country of origin?

6. Voice

- What tone of voice do you use in your country?
- What is considered polite and what is considered rude?
- What does sarcasm or humor sound like in your culture?

7. "Speak" the following in gestures.

- What time is it?
- I have a stomachache.
- Goodbye.
- It's too hot.
- That's too loud.
- Go away. Scram!
- Ouch!
- Can I have a turn?
- What's up?
- It's over there.
- I'm leaving.
- He's crazy!
- Stop!
- Come in, please.
- You're late! [pointing to wristwatch]

8. Media: Scrutinizing people in the media is an excellent way to observe and learn nonverbal communication patterns specific to American culture.

- Observe nonverbal communication and body language of media personalities, newscasters, and talk show hosts.
- Examine how they change their facial expressions from one situation to another.

9. Charades

- Playing the game of Charades helps you open up and not be reserved about nonverbal or body language.

10. Body language

- Observe what people do with different body parts and facial features—head, eyes, eyebrows, mouth, nose, chin, and so on. Record your observations as accurately as you can, and indicate what you think these facial expressions mean.

- Observe how close together people from different countries stand next to each other in various settings—in line at the ticket counter, at the office, in the ball park, at a restaurant, and so on.

- Observe how people use touch in relationships with acquaintances, colleagues, family, friends, and strangers.

11. Other observations

- Feel free to add other observations you may witness during your professional and social interactions. Record these observations as accurately as you can, indicating what each of these expressions may mean.

11

Pronunciation: Eloquently Speaking

Even if you have taken English as a second language (ESL) classes for several years, you may have realized that your conversational English still does not sound the same as that of a native speaker. Probably you've been focusing on vocabulary and specifics of theory, so your study has not addressed the subtleties of conversational English that give the language its style. This chapter introduces you to various time-tested approaches to fine-tuning your pronunciation that emphasize how words actually *sound* in rapid spoken English, rather than rules for pronunciation based on spelling. With use of these approaches, together with pronunciation practice drills to overcome specific error sound patterns, you can expect very noticeable improvement in the clarity and overall quality of your conversational English.

As an ESL learner, you may sometimes wonder whether it's really necessary to sound like a native speaker. Is "perfection" in a second language a requirement for enjoying yourself socially or for your job performance? Isn't it enough to achieve a level of fluency and clarity that's more than adequate to make your message under-

stood? And can traces of your original "foreign" accent have any significant effect on the clarity and intelligibility of your English?

For any second language speaker, ongoing self-assessment along with drills and creative practice sessions is essential for foreign accent management. The skills and strategies presented in this chapter are tools to make this lifelong process easier and more satisfying. So approach this aspect of accent management with determination and discipline to achieve and maintain clarity, not with frustration and feelings of failure to attain perfection.

What Is Pronunciation?

The act of *pronunciation* is a means whereby the organs of speech, the articulators, combine the speech sounds to form words of adequate intelligibility. These words are put together in a quick sequence in order to convey a message. The act of pronunciation leads to rapid spoken English—conversational speech.

When you began learning the pronunciation of each English word, you probably made a list of practice words that were more difficult for you. Then you sounded out each of the alphabetic characters in the word according to the way it was spelled. Most ESL learners rely on spelling for pronunciation, blissfully unaware of the numerous "exceptions" to the rules of spelling in English: the silent e, "i before e," and so on. Consequently, most pronunciation problems stem from the fact that the English language is *unphonetic*—words are not always pronounced the way they are spelled.

Being able to pronounce the words correctly in isolation does not mean you can get it "correct" in connected speech. You may have noticed that even after you've just been through an excellent practice session with word lists, the minute you start talking to a colleague, the words don't sound as clear as they did in practice. This is because when the words combine into running speech, several factors (see below) can have specific effects on pronunciation of individual word segments.

Factors That Affect Pronunciation

Pronunciation in running speech is influenced by:

- syllable stress
- omission or addition of speech sounds
- combining sounds between words to create a whole new sound unit

These changes, which may occur *within* or *between* words in fast fluent speech, have developed into specific features within spoken English. Different linguistics experts may subcategorize these changes or just list them as exceptions to pronunciation. Accent coaches, however, may sometimes reorganize and classify these features for a simplified system of pronunciation to suit their clientele.

We can all agree that attention to spelling is essential for written language. But to master pronunciation, it is more practical to listen carefully to the way people actually speak, than to relate pronunciation to spelling for every single word. No doubt you have already discovered that phonetic transcription exercises (refer back to Chapter 4) are more useful than the "English spelling" to identify actual speech sounds present within a word for correct pronunciation. Using phonetic transcription symbols will help to reduce pronunciation mishaps.

As discussed in earlier chapters, your pronunciation skills are affected by the structure and rules of your native language. Every language in the world has a set of rules for spelling, pronunciation, grammar, and so on. Keeping in mind the organizational rules of your native language, you must train yourself to differentiate them from the rules of English, and to assess its influence on your spoken English. This awareness is the key to reducing the influence of your native pronunciation and replacing it with the English equivalent in this process of foreign accent management.

Some people may assume that reducing the influence of your native language rules to learn English is a direct link to forgetting your own language and perhaps even your culture. Is it possible to retain your native language rules and learn new rules too? Absolutely! If becoming proficient in a new language and its accent is something you need professionally and socially, then there is no question you must pursue a program such as foreign accent management.

Because culture is so intertwined with language, we go through an adjustment phase in which we get habituated to doing things a different way, not necessarily "our" way or "their" way. The point is that culture undergoes its own transformation periodically, whether you or I take an active part in it or not. Undoubtedly, we all are involved in the culture transformation and globalization that is happening around the world right now. We shall realize our part in it only in hindsight.

Moreover, pronunciation has a direct effect on accents. If you can pronounce a word correctly both in isolation and within sentences (in conversation), then you probably are using the "correct" accent. Now that you are becoming aware of other factors that influence pronunciation in running speech, the same factors affect accent also. This chapter's pronunciation exercises will take you through a process to achieve clarity of spoken language, but you may still retain traces of your native language accent.

Correcting Pronunciation

As is evident from the array of language classes, audio foreign language learning tapes, and accent improvement programs available, there are many ways to correct pronunciation in a second language. Various professionals—accent coaches, speech therapists, teachers, and so on—will use certain basic guidelines to begin the process of correcting pronunciation. In addition, they will incorporate other techniques and strategies that they have found through other resources, research, and personal experience.

As mentioned earlier, the approach to pronunciation improvement presented in this chapter is a time-tested method that is sure to transform the clarity of your speech if you put in dedicated practice. This approach includes specific techniques and strategies that I have adopted in my own practice and used in concert with vowel and consonant drills. After experimenting with each of them in conversa-

tions with friends and colleagues and receiving constructive feedback, the clarity of my speech improved immensely. (And I was able to hone the skill of accent switching and get it right nearly 50 percent of the time.)

In addition to vowel and consonant drills (presented in the worksheet at the end of the chapter five and six), training in correct pronunciation incorporated in this book's approach to accent management includes but is not restricted to the following:

- differentiating between English spelling and pronunciation through International Phonetic Alphabet (IPA) transcription

- breaking down words into units called syllables and listening to how they combine within words

- understanding the influences of weaker or stronger speech sounds within and between words (deletions, add-ons, and assimilation)

- other pronunciation variations: presence and absence of aspiration, stress variations, suffix "-ed" endings, medial /t/ as in "bitten" and "water," others

You already are familiar with use of the IPA from earlier chapters and probably have become aware of just how often English spelling does not match pronunciation. Read along further to understand more about the other items listed in training pronunciation, beginning with syllables.

Syllables

As defined in Chapter 9, syllables are units of spoken language that is larger than a segment but smaller than a word and made up of speech sounds in various combinations. Even though English is a stressed language (rather than a syllable-timed language; refer back to Chapter 9), it may be useful to understand how syllables are grouped and relate them to the stress placement within words.

Sometimes the syllables are hard to identify, because they may not be clearly enunciated. For example, in adjacent syllables when two vowels appear, as in "do/ing," the word is pronounced with a single muscular movement, even though it can be grouped into two syllables. Other similar words are "meteor," and "neonate."

Syllable Workout

Identifying the number of syllables in a given word will assist in pronunciation. For easier practice, these syllable units can be recognized and numbered. Words can be grouped into those with one, two, three, or multiple syllables Accordingly, they are termed monosyllabic, bisyllabic, trisyllabic, and multisyllabic words.

Practice saying the following monosyllabic, bisyllabic, trisyllabic, and multisyllabic words aloud. Use your critical listening skills to hear each of the syllables clearly. Although you may be enunciating each of the syllables in word practice drills, these syllables may undergo either subtle or more obvious changes in combination with other words in running speech (demonstrated later in the chapter).

Monosyllabic words

an	to	three	bite	sit	hill
1	1	1	1	1	1

way	speech
1	1

Bisyllabic words

apron	orange	eaten	sister
a/pron	o/range	ea/ten	sis/ter
1 2	1 2	1 2	1 2

divide
di/vide
1 2

Trisyllabic words

develop	construction
de/ve/lop	cons/truc/tion
1 2 3	1 2 3

management
ma/nage/ment
1   2   3

Multisyllabic words

conversation	hippopotamus
con/ver/sa/tion	hip/po/po/ta/mus
1 2 3 4	1 2 3 4 5

parapsychology	intelligibility
pa/ra/psy/cho/lo/gy	in/te/lli/gi/bi/li/ty
1 2 3 4 5 6	1 2 3 4 5 6 7

Syllables and Pronunciation

In order to relate syllables to correct pronunciation, the aspect of stress within the words must be considered. When an English word has more than one syllable, one of the syllables must be stressed. In Chapter 9 we saw that the position of the stress is almost invariably fixed for each word. ESL students *must* learn the position of this stress in order to identify the correct pronunciation.

Monosyllabic and bisyllabic words are fairly easy to pronounce. However, pronunciation challenges that affect intelligibility generally are quick to be noticed in trisyllabic and multisyllabic words. Here is a simple process that has worked consistently for some of my students: First, identify and number the syllables. Then decide which syllables go together based on the stress patterns—primary, secondary, and weak (refer to Chapter 9). This will point you to the correct pronunciation.

Let's review the process:

Example: develop

Number of syllables: de/ve/lop = 3. (So it's a trisyllabic word.) Now number the syllables:

de   ve   lop
1   2   3

Stress pattern: The middle syllable, **ve**, has the primary stress; **de** has secondary stress; and **lop** has the weak stress.

Pronunciation: Syllables 1 and 2 go together in quick sequence, to get to the primary stress on syllable 2. Syllable 3 follows to complete the word. So the pronunciation is **deve̲lop**.

Practice saying this combination aloud multiple times. More exercises are provided in the worksheet at the end of the chapter.

Important Exceptions

In some two-syllable words, the stress is on the *first* syllable for a *noun* and on the *second* syllable for a *verb*. It is important to recognize the change in meaning resulting from the change in position of the stress. Table 11–1 lists some examples.

Here are some example sentences using words listed in Table 11–1 that highlight the different meanings with syllable stress variation.

- ob**ject**—verb: We *object* to your decision.
- **ob**ject—noun: What is the name of this *object*?
- re**cord**—verb: Are you planning to *record* the speech?
- **re**cord—noun: They have no *record* of your application.

In addition, similar-sounding words such as "accept," "aspect," "except," and so on can be very confusing to many second language students. The meaning of each of these words can be understood only from the context in which it is used. Sometimes

Table 11–1. Two-Syllable Words in Which Stress Changes Meaning

Noun Form	Verb Form
record	re**cord**
convict	con**vict**
rebel	re**bel**
progress	pro**gress**
pervert	per**vert**
import	im**port**
address	ad**dress**
research	re**search**
protest	pro**test**
object	ob**ject**

a speaker who is aware of a word's meaning may nevertheless mispronounce the word, either by mistake or because of lack of awareness of cultural/dialectical differences (as in "ask" versus "aks"). Some examples follow:

- aspect—noun: Which *aspect* of the project am I responsible for?
- accept—verb: We *accept* this challenge of foreign accent management.
- except—preposition: Everyone came *except* her best friend.
- exception—noun: We'll make an *exception* in your case.
- expect—verb: What did you *expect* from the seminar?
- affect—verb: How did the downsizing *affect* you?
- effect—noun: What was the *effect* of the chemotherapy on your aunt?
- affect—noun: His general *affect* suggested he was very depressed.

Sometimes the similarity in the sound of such words confuses the ESL student into assuming that they share similar meanings as well, so the student tends to use them interchangeably, despite the differences in their meanings. This creates confusion for the listener and affects the comprehension of the message. Thus, using syllable stress will assist in deciding on the correct pronunciation, thereby increasing the clarity of your speech.

Adopting Weaker Articulation

Words, especially those that express grammatical relationships such as and, had, them, etc., are particularly affected during a fast-paced conversation. Some words take on stronger stress when pronounced in isolation or may become weaker in the midst of running speech or conversation. Try pronouncing the following example words in isolation or with emphasis and then within phrases or sentences:

In isolation or with emphasis	Within phrase or sentence
and	this and that = this **n** that (notice that the word "and" is shortened to just "n")
a	This is **a** pencil. (referring to the object) This is a pencil. (referring to number of the object—not 2 or 3 pencils but only 1)
had	He had gone with him. = He'**d** gone with him.

him	with him = with'**im** (**h** is eliminated)
not	did not = didn't
(in contractions)	will not = won't
them	mash them = mash'**em** show them = show'**em**
-ing	What's **goin'** on? (the g is dropped in casual use—doin', happenin') *versus* Are you **going**? (the g is *not* dropped on a stressed word)

Use the worksheet exercises at the end of the chapter to practice adopting weaker articulation within your sentences. Practice multiple times before attempting to experiment on your friends or colleagues who are native speakers. With little or no practice, your speech may come across as feeble, or your articulation sounds may seem unnatural to a native speaker. In addition, your attempts to practice any of these pronunciation exceptions or rules may sound unnatural to your family or friends of similar ethnicity—they are used to your native language—accented English, and anything different may be jarring, inviting accusatory comments such as "You are putting on an accent!"

Deletions

The term *deletion* implies that some speech units are completely dropped, especially when they occur as a part of a cluster of consonants. In English conversation, alveolar consonant sounds—t and d—at the ends of words normally are dropped, and initial weak vowels may be omitted, as in the examples in Table 11–2.

Other Deletions

Deletions are more common with speech units that occur as a part of a cluster of consonants. There are certain words in the English language that are called *high-frequency words*—words used often in everyday conversation. When these high-frequency words precede other words (typically auxiliary or "helping" verbs) such as "did," "will," "is," "could," or "should," in a question format, they undergo changes in their speech units. The high-frequency words are:

- the /h/ family words: "he," "her," "his," "him," "hers'
- "have" used as a helping verb ("**Have** you eaten breakfast yet?" "I **have** not made any mistakes with my drills so far.")

For example, the words "Did he" in the question "Did he go to the prom?" become **did'e**—/h/ is essentially dropped and the e sound is merged with the preceding word. The following sections address these deletions in detail, with examples.

he/her Deletions

Pronunciation is affected within quick-paced conversation when /h/ from "he" or /h/ from "her" is deleted and the remaining syllable is merged with the preceding word, as in the following examples.

- "**Did he** leave town again?" /h/ is deleted to make the sentence sound like "**Did'e** leave town again?"
- "**Didn't he** know we were coming at four?" /h/ is deleted to make the sentence sound like "**Didn'e** know we were coming at four?"
- "**Will her** office be moved to the new building?" /h/ is deleted to make the sentence sound like "**Will'er** office be moved to the new building?"
- "**Did her** boss agree with the proposal?" /h/ is deleted to make the sentence sound like "**Did'er** boss agree with the proposal?"

The key is to practice saying these sentences aloud to hear the deletions within running speech. By identifying the differences between written language and spoken language, you gain an important realization as an ESL learner: you cannot transfer the sentence drills in your tutorials exactly into

Table 11–2. Deletion of Speech Sounds

Alveolar Consonants	Initial Weak Vowels	
next day = nex day	go away = go way	try again = try gain
mashed potatoes = mash potatoes	**Silent Consonants**	
stopped speaking = stop speaking	listen = lisen	thumb = thum
last time = las time	answer = anser	isle = ile
last chance = las chance	walk = wak (long a)	Sioux City = Su City
left turn = lef turn	palm = pam	often = offen
kept quiet = kep quiet	thistle = thisel	climb = clim
postman = pos man		

conversational speech. The worksheet at the end of the chapter contains additional examples for your practice.

Deletions in "have" Helping Verbs

Pronunciation is affected when /ha/ from the word "have" is deleted and the final e, being silent, is replaced and modified as /ve/ or /uv/. Notice that these "condensed" phonetic forms, used in rapidly spoken English, are not the same as a *contraction*. (Contractions are shortened forms acceptable in less formal speech or language, as in written dialogue—for example, *can't* for "cannot," *won't* for "will not.") Review the modifications within the words in the following list.

> could have = could'**uv**
> couldn't have = couldn'**uv**
>
> would have = would'**uv**
> wouldn't have = wouldn'**uv**
>
> should have = should'**uv**
> shouldn't have = shouldn'**u**
>
> must have = must'**uv**
> mustn't have = mustn'**uv**

Now listen to the pronunciation of these words within sentences in the following examples. Practice saying both versions of the sentences aloud to critically listen to differences in pronunciation.

- "You **could have** called the office for an appointment." /ha/ from the word "have" is deleted, to make the sentence sound like "You **could'uv** called the office for an appointment."

- "You **couldn't have** completed this project so quickly!" /ha/ from the word "have" is deleted to make the sentence sound like "You **couldn'tuv** completed this project so quickly!"

- "I **would have** called yesterday, but I couldn't." /ha/ from the word "have" is deleted to make the

sentence sound like "I **would'uv** called yesterday, but I couldn't."

- "I **wouldn't have** changed the plans so soon." /ha/ from the word "have" is deleted to make the sentence sound like "I **wouldn'tuv** changed the plans so soon."

- "I **should have** returned this book yesterday." /ha/ from the word "have" is deleted to make the sentence sound like "I **should'uv** returned the book yesterday."

- "This project **shouldn't have** been so difficult!" /ha/ from the word "have" is deleted to make the sentence sound like "This project **shouldn'tuv** been so difficult."

- "You **must have** been mistaken about your boss." /ha/ from the word "have" is deleted to make the sentence sound like "You **must'uv** been mistaken."

- "He **mustn't** have done that." /ha/ from the word "have" is deleted to make the sentence sound like "He **musn'tuv** have done that."

- "Things **might have** turned out differently for Bob." /ha/ from the word "have" is deleted to make the sentence sound like "Things **might'uv** turned out differently for Bob."

Again, refer to the worksheet for more practice sentences.

Add-ons

The term *add-on* implies that a sound or a syllable is attached to the original word in rapid spoken English. The most common add-on is related to the use of "is" and "isn't" in coordination with /h/ words such as "he," "her," "his," hers." Notice that although the words "is" and "isn't" are spelled with the letter s, they are pronounced with the sound /z/.

Next, as in previous deletions, /h/ is deleted in the combination of "is" and "he" to give "is'e." The written form—as in a sentence—appears as "Is 'e here yet?" In the following examples, however, careful listening will reveal that besides the deletion of /h/, the phoneme /z/ is "added on" or replaces /s/ in most of the "is" and "isn't" combinations. This family of add-ons is summarized in the following list:

is he	=	**iz'e**
isn't he	=	**izn'e**
is her	=	**iz'er**
isn't he	=	**izn'er**
is his	=	**iz'iz**
isn't hi	=	**izn'iz**

These words are used in the following example sentences. Practice saying both versions of the sentences aloud to hear the differences in pronunciation.

- "**Is he** coming home soon?" /h /from "he" is dropped, and /s/ from "Is" is replaced or modifies to /z/. Now the sentence sounds like "**Iz'e** coming home soon?"

- "**Isn't he** coming to visit today?" As in the preceding example, /s/ is replaced or modified to /z/, and /h/ from "he" is dropped. Now the sentence sounds like "**Izn'e** coming to visit today?

- "**Is his** home in Philadelphia?" /h/ is dropped from "his," and /s/ from "Is" and "his" is replaced by /z/, forming the modified sentence "**Iz'iz** home in Philadelphia?"

- "**Isn't his** manager Mr. Smith?" /h/ is dropped from "his," and /s/ in "Isn't" and "his" is replaced by /z/,

forming the modified sentence "**Izn'iz** manager Mr. Smith?"

- "**Is her** sister engaged?" /h/ is deleted, /z/ is added, so the sentence sounds like "**Iz'er** sister engaged?"

- "**Isn't her** apartment cozy?" /h/ is deleted, /z/ is added, so the sentence sounds like "**Izn'er** apartment cozy?"

"You" Add-on

Another add-on to be considered is the word "you." "You" is not completely deleted as with /h/ words in the previous sections. The vowel sound in "you" may be shortened to a schwa (ə) or otherwise modified in certain cases: The emphasis on "you" is greater if the speaker wants to focus on *you*, the person. If the emphasis is not necessary, "you" is a weak word in the message and therefore is shortened slightly in conversation.

Pronunciation is affected when "you" is preceded by a verb in different forms:

- Verbs that end in a vowel, as in "do you," are shortened to a schwa: **do yə** (IPA)

- Verbs in negative contractions, as in "don't you" (voiceless alveolar), also are modified: **don' tʃu** (IPA) ("don'chu")

- Verbs that end in voiced alveolar consonants, as in "did you," also are modified: **did dʒ u** (IPA) ("did'ju")

Now study the following list.

do you	=	**do yə**
will you	=	**will yə**
don't you	=	**don'tʃu**
didn't you	=	**didn'tʃu**
did you	=	**did dʒu**
had you	=	**had dʒu**

These words are used in the following example sentences. Practice saying both versions of the sentences aloud to listen to the differences in pronunciation.

- "How **do you** feel?" "ou" is deleted and replaced by /ə/ (schwa); now the sentence sounds like "How **do yə** feel?"

- "**Will you** be coming over?" "ou" is deleted and replaced by /ə/ (schwa); now the sentence sounds like "**Will yə** be coming over?"

- "**Don't you** want to come over?" "you" is deleted and replaced by /tʃu/; now the sentence sounds like "**Don't tʃu** want to come over?"

- "**Didn't you** bake the cake yesterday?" "you" is deleted and replaced by /tʃu/; now the sentence sounds like "**Didn't tʃu** bake the cake yesterday?"

- "**Won't you** at least come by for a few minutes?" "you" is deleted and replaced by /tʃu/; now the sentence sounds like "**Wont' tʃu** at least come by for a few minutes?"

- "**Hadn't you** called for a meeting last week?" "you" is deleted and replaced by /tʃu/; now the sentence sounds like "**Hadn't tʃu** called for a meeting last week?"

- "**Shouldn't you** be taking your medicines?" "you" is deleted and replaced by /tʃu/; now the sentence sounds like "**Shouldn't tʃu** be taking your medicines?"

- "**Wouldn't you** like to go?" "you" is deleted and replaced by /tʃu/; now the sentence sounds like "**Wouldn't tʃu** like to go?"

- "**Couldn't you** call your parents for permission?" "you" is deleted and replaced by /tʃu/; now the sentence sounds like "**Couldn't tʃu** call your parents for permission?"

- "**Did you** have to cancel your appointment?" "you" is deleted and replaced by /dʒu/; now the sentence sounds like "**Did dʒu** have to cancel your appointment?"

- "**Had you** ever gone bowling before?" "you" is deleted and replaced by /dʒu/; now the sentence sounds like "**Had dʒu** ever gone bowling before?"

- "**Would you** like a take-out menu?" "you" is deleted and replaced by /dʒu/; now the sentence sounds like "**Would dʒu** like a takeout menu?"

- "**Should you** be coming in on weekends?" "you" is deleted and replaced by /dʒu/; now the sentence sounds like "**Should dʒu** be coming in on weekends?"

- "**Could you** meet with the committee tomorrow?" "you" is deleted and replaced by /dʒu/; now the sentence sounds like "**Could dʒu** meet the committee tomorrow?"

More practice sentences are listed in the worksheet at the end of the chapter.

Assimilation

Deletions and add-ons aren't the only ways in which speech sounds can change in rapid conversational English. Some speech sound units tend to change character altogether, because adjacent sounds frequently influence each other within sentences. They tend to become more alike, or assimilate. This process of *assimilation* also is called *linking* by linguists and phoneticians alike. Linking refers to the blending of the end of one word with the beginning of the next, so that no real separation between the two words can be heard.

The boundary between two speech sounds is difficult to represent within conversation. The stronger speech sound influences the weaker sound, and the speech structure anticipates the next move that causes the linking or assimilation to occur. Native speakers of many languages typically do not realize that they link words all the time within conversations using the manner of speech that is most natural to them. So a reasonable assumption is that running speech in most languages undergoes changes in structure or modifications of speech sounds without changing the meaning of the message conveyed.

An important distinction is that assimilation occurs in rapid informal speech, not during formal or slow speech. It is "heard," not "seen"—the spelling of the word remains the same. Because assimilation is not represented in a word's spelling, many non-native speakers are skeptical. They may interpret the speech sound changes as carelessness on the part of the speaker, until they understand the presence of cultural idiosyncrasies and accept the grammatical exceptions as "normal" in everyday speech. As we do with other features of spoken English, it is useful to listen to the way people actually speak, rather than trying to correlate each syllable of every word with the English spelling.

Assimilation has been categorized in various ways by different linguists and researchers. A general classification is presented here, with examples. Begin by practicing the example words and phrases in isolation, and then progress to their use within sentences to understand the influence of assimilation in making conversational speech fluent.

1. *Anticipatory assimilation*: A sound is influenced by a following sound, as in "ten bikes" = tem bikes. Try making sentences with the following examples:

- handbag   = ham bag   nd > m
- mean bark = meam bark
- lean beef   = leam beef
- good bye   = goob bye   d > b
- good girl   = goog girl   d > g

2. *Progressive assimilation*: The sound is influenced by the preceding sound, as in "that guard" = that kuard.
- that boy = that poy   t > p
- that girl = that kirl   t > k

3. *Reciprocal assimilation* demonstrates existence of mutual influence or fusion of sounds, as in "tennis shoes" = tennishoes.
- this shop = thishop   s > sh
- this shoe = thishoe

4. *Exact assimilation* is noted when the last consonant of a word is the same as the first consonant of the following word, we usually pronounce that sound only once, thereby linking the two words. For example: "Call the main number." Here are a few more examples.
- nine nickels
- cheap paper

Using these and other similar examples in sentences and saying them aloud will help you recognize the assimilation in your own speech. Refer to the worksheet for additional practice.

5. *Connector assimilation*: Words that begin with a vowel are linked or fixed to a preceding consonant, as in "I'm eating an apple." With assimilation, the sentence reads as follows: "I'meating a napple." Make sentences with the following examples and practice saying them aloud.
- an acorn   = an nacorn
- nine apples = nine napples

Other Variations Affecting Pronunciation of Rapid Spoken English

Aspiration on /p/ and /k/

The English speech sounds /p, b, k, g, t, d, θ, and ð/ do not have aspirated and unaspirated counterparts. Researchers have grouped /p, b/, /k, g/, and other speech sounds as minimal pairs and differentiated them according to various characteristics such as presence or absence of voicing, air flow, and other distinctive features related to linguistics, phonetics, or speech pathology. A few of these features, as appropriate, have been discussed in the chapters on vowels and consonants.

Some languages on the Asian subcontinent (Sanskrit, Hindi, and others), however, have speech sounds broken down into aspirated and unaspirated sounds. For example /p/ sound has two variations: /p/ unaspirated, with no air puff when the lips are released, and the /p-uh/ with aspiration, with an air puff when the lips are released. The other sound in this minimal pair, /b/, has the same variations: /b/ unaspirated and /b-uh/ with aspiration.

Similar variations are attributed to each of the other speech sounds for minimal pairs. Therefore, an ESL speaker whose native language is Hindi or any other language often does not recognize the need to use an aspirated /p/ sound for the word "pen." The same error speech sound is used with /k/ for "car," /t/ for "tape," and /θ/ for "think."

Working with students from different countries whose languages ranged from Spanish, French, German, and Swedish to Korean, Mandarin, Arabic, and Swahili, I have noticed similar difficulties among ESL learners in distinguishing between and using aspirated and unaspirated sounds (or a lack of awareness of aspirated versus unaspirated sounds), or sometimes inappropriate placement of aspiration (on /b/ or /g/ instead of /p/ or /k/). So depending on your country of origin, you may need more or less practice with this aspect of pronunciation.

Practice the words in Table 11–3 with aspiration.

Use the target speech sounds presented in the worksheet for Chapter 6, on consonants, for more practice on aspiration.

Stress Variations

Although Chapter 9, on intonation, addresses stress variations in detail, a brief mention to tie it to running speech seems appropriate. Conversational or running speech is affected immensely by rhythm and stress. The most important words in a message usually are enunciated using precise articulation and emphasized with intonation and stress. This emphasis is to help the listener focus on the essential points of the message. However, the remainder of the message is hastened or shortened with fading intonation-level markers.

Table 11–3. Aspirated Consonant Sounds

/p/	/k/	/t/	/ð/
Paul	coward	temper	thought
pot	computer	tabulate	therapy
program	barbecue	trainer	throw
department	corporate	teacher	thorough
composite	curriculum	template	through

As an ESL learner, you must recognize and understand the relationship of stressed and unstressed or weak syllables and words if you want your spoken English to sound like the natural, conversational English you hear every day. To decide between stressed and unstressed words, you must classify them as lexical or grammatical words. Recall from Chapter Nine that they also are referred to as content and function words.

Example 1

It was the best vacation house for us to lease.

In this sentence, certain words carry the stress, because they carry the meaning of the sentence. Hence they convey the message to the listener. These words are considered "strong" words and are termed lexical or content words. Lexical words are nouns, verbs, adjectives, and adverbs.

The remaining words act as connectors between the lexical words and are called grammatical or function words. They are unstressed or weak. The grammatical words are conjunctions, pronouns, prepositions, and auxiliary (helping) verbs.

Example 2

It was the best vacation house for us to lease.

The underlined words are lexical words—strong words that carry the message of the sentence. The other words are grammatical connector words. Now read the sentence aloud, the first time without any stress and a second time stressing the underlined phrases. Notice the difference in your articulation of the stressed words and the ease of conveying the meaning correctly. (Refer to the worksheet for Chapter 9 for more practice on intonation.)

The Schwa (ə) Factor

One important feature to remember is that in all weak or unstressed forms, the schwa vowel sound, ə, is used. The unstressed schwa, ə, often intrudes between a stressed vowel and following /l/ or /r/ speech sound. Although it is not represented in the spelling, the sound is critical to correct pronunciation and hence is represented in phonetic transcription as in the following examples.

- "eel": ɨəl
- "sour": saʊər

This schwa vowel sound, ə, is difficult to detect. If you think there is a vowel sound within a word but you are unsure, it probably is the schwa. The word "pool," for example, is transcribed phonetically as **puəl**. Most ESL speakers are unable to detect the presence of the schwa vowel sound and hence omit the sound. The word may sound like **pul** without the schwa vowel sound.

A few more examples are listed in Table 11–4. It is important to transcribe these words phonetically before attempting their pronunciation.

Table 11–4. Transcribing the Schwa

English Spelling	IPA	English Spelling	IPA	English Spelling	IPA
steal	stɨəl	steel	stɨəl	tour	tuər
fool	fuəl	teal	tɨəl	sour	saʊər

Suffixes "-ed"

How does a suffix relate to pronunciation? A suffix is a morphological unit of speech that is attached to the *end* of words and carries grammatical meaning; a suffix changes the *structure* of the word without altering the fundamental part of speech.

Pronunciation of suffixes changes depending on the phonological influence within which they occur. The "-ed"' denoting regular past tense is pronounced /ed/ after /t/ and /d/ (alveolar consonants), as in "wanted" and "added." However, it is pronounced /d/ after all other voiced sounds, as in "sprayed," "clubbed," and "hanged." And it is pronounced /t/ after voiceless sounds, as in "worked," "passed," and "benched."

A few examples are listed in Table 11–5. More practice words are included in the worksheet at the end of the chapter.

Medial /t/ Sound

Many ESL learners find it difficult to bring a natural accent to words with medial /t/, as in "button" and "bitten." This speech sound has two different variations; one variation of /t/ sounds like /ʌ/ as in "up," and the other sounds like /d/ as in "dog."

Many students tend to pronounce medial /t/ with too much force, making the word sound somewhat harsh to the ears. If necessary, refer back to the /t/ exercises from the worksheet in Chapter 6, on consonants. Which articulators come together to pro-

duce this phoneme? The tongue or the lingua strikes the tip behind the front teeth to produce the /t/ sound. Some ESL learners assume that with a double "tt," as in the word "button," both phonemes must be articulated—so they overstress the sound by striking the tongue harder behind the teeth.

For example, if you listen to those who speak any of the languages or its dialects from India, you will notice pronunciation hard on /t/ not only in the medial position ("button") but also in the final position ("forget"). This is because they are used to pronouncing the /t/ sound clearly in their native language without changing or reducing the strength of articulation. This speech pattern of their native language affects the pronunciation, so /t/ in the word "button" is very loud and harsh sounding.

Now let's proceed to how medial /t/ should actually be produced in English conversational speech.

Medial /t/ Sound, as in "bitten"

Within certain words, the medial /t/ is shortened to stop its complete release as /t/ and changes to a sound like /ʌ/. This can be explained according to the place of articulation. The point of contact for /t/ is the tongue tip behind the front teeth—the alveolar ridge. This contact point shifts to a point toward the back to the throat, as in /ʌ/, and then is followed by /n/ to complete the word. The actual sound assumes the shortened form of "un." Selective listening and auditory discrimination are essential to

Table 11–5. Pronunciation of "-ed" Suffixes

Final t plus /ed/	Final d (or de) plus /ed/	Voiceless: /t/	Voiced: /d/
tooted	plodded	coughed	moaned
pouted	jaded	forked	starred

hear the sound transition clearly. The same rule applies within compound words.

For example, say the word "bitten," pronouncing /t/ with aspiration. Now say it by shortening the /t/ sound and completing the word with /n/ sound: "bitten" = **bitn**.

Now review the following examples, presented with both English spellings and IPA transcriptions. Practice saying them aloud both ways, first with the hard /t/ sound and then with /ʌ/ sound followed by /n/. Refer to the worksheet at the end of the chapter for more practice words.

English Spelling	IPA Transcription— within Conversation
button	bʌtn = butn
fatten	fætn = fatn
kitten	kɪtn = kitn

Medial /t/ Sound as in "water"

Within other words, the medial /t/ changes to sound like /d/. The point of contact remains the same (behind the front teeth, on the alveolar ridge); however, the voicing is changed. The voiceless /t/ changes to sound like its voiced counterpart, /d/. The actual sound is somewhere between the /t/ and the /d/ sounds. Selective listening and auditory discrimination are essential to hear the sound clearly. The same rule applies within compound words.

For example, say the word "water" with very clear pronunciation of /t/. Now say the word quickly, changing /t/ to voiced /d/: "waw-der." Place a hand on your throat to detect the change of voicing between the /t/ and the /d/ sound when you say the word "water" = **wadɚ**. However, it is important to remember that the /d/ sound should *not* be exaggerated but is pronounced lightly and quickly. Review the examples in Table 11–6, which presents both the English spelling and the phonetic (IPA) transcription.

Table 11–6. Medial /t/ Sounds

English Spelling	IPA—within Conversation
city	sɪti = sɪdi
butter	bʌtɚ = bʌdɚ
attic	ætɪk = æddɪk

Idiosyncrasies of e

Final e Variations

In the following words, /e /is pronounced /i/ in "beat" or /ɛ/ as in "bed."

- knee /i/
- seven /ɛ/
- Resume /ɛ/
- Sesame /i/

Silent e

When /e/ is added at the end of the word, the pronunciation of the word changes: Short vowels usually change to long vowels, as in the example sentences in the next paragraph. Most second language learners initially are not aware of this change. Sometimes the ESL speaker finds out the hard way: Mispronouncing what seemed to be the correct word results in another word with an entirely different meaning. Silent e not only changes the vowel sound from short to long but also creates a *different* word.

In the following two sentences, it's easy to see the effect of a silent e:

1. What did you bring for a *snake*/snack?
2. Please *tack*/take a seat.

More practice words are provided in the worksheet at the end of the chapter.

The u Variations

The silent e rules also apply to certain words spelled with u. Depending on whether the word ends with a silent e, the meaning of the word will differ. And it is essential to use the right word to convey the right meaning within a message. Variations in the pronunciation of u parallel those for a. Review the u variations in the examples listed in Table 11–7.

Final "-ous" Pronunciation

When there are two or more vowels in a word such as "beat," the preceding vowel takes the lead in its pronunciation. However, in words with "-ous" endings, the final vowel sound is pronounced /ʌs/, with /ʌ/ as in the word "us"—the vowel sound, /u/, takes the lead. The o and u sounds are not pronounced individually and are not rounded to "ow" as in the word "bout." For example, the word "famous" is transcribed phonetically as **femʌs** and hence is pronounced "famus." On the other hand, because of its final e, the word "mouse" is transcribed phonetically as **maʊs** and hence is pronounced "mous." Refer to the worksheet at the end of the chapter for more practice.

Summary

Attention to all of the features of rapidly spoken English discussed in this chapter will definitely help to make you sound more natural and fluent in conversation. Although such features are considered to be important characteristics of normal spoken English, they may not be represented in basic spelling or included in ESL tutorials for beginners. They typically are overlooked until you realize that your conversational English does not sound the same as the native speaker's.

As you focus your practice on each of the error sound patterns, it is important to practice each one in isolation to identify the syllable stress. But it then becomes essential to proceed to pronunciation within structured sentences and listen to how the features change (through deletions, add-ons, and so on) in rapid speech or within conversation.

Table 11–7. The u Variations

but	brute	mutt	mute
rut	ruse	flutter	flute
putt	put	bug	bugle

WORKSHEET 11

Pronunciation Practice

Syllable Identification/Stress Transcription/Numbering

Syllable Identification

Identify the number of syllables. Repeat this exercise several times until you are comfortable in recognizing and identifying the syllables in each of the words. Tap out the syllables on the table as you say them *aloud* to hear the correct number of syllables.

Syllable Identification	Number of Syllables	Your List of Words	Number of Syllables
tight	1		
seat			
beverage			
acorn			
contribution			
direction			
transportation			
California			
retrospect			
blemishes			
punctuality			
interpretation			
interrogation			
equipment			
larynx			

Syllable and Stress Transcription

Divide each word into its syllables and identify the stress for each one. Then write each of the syllables in the appropriate stress pattern column. Primary stress can be indicated by an underscore (__). Secondary stress can be indicated by the symbol ^. Weak stress can be indicated by *. The first word has been done for you.

English Spelling	Syllable Identification	Primary Stress	Secondary Stress	Weak or No Stress
commission	*com <u>mis</u> sion^	mi	ssion	com
library				
Pennsylvania				
compassionate				
shadow				
outrageous				
advertisement				
wasteful				
stationary				
inspection				
capital				
sincere				
choreography				
Montessori				
Tylenol				
management				

Syllable Numbering

Identify and number the syllables in the following words. Tap out the syllables on the table as you combine the right numbers and <u>say them aloud</u>. This will help you achieve the correct pronunciation. Practice multiple times and ask for clarification whenever necessary from anyone well versed in the pronunciation of English. The first word has been done for you.

Syllable Identification	Number of Syllables	Stress Patterns
<u>ban</u>quet^ 1 2	2	primary (1): **ban** secondary (2): **quet**
dictionary		
championship		
identification		
intelligibility		
beginner		
adaptability		
rhinoceros		
prevalent		
quintuplet		
triplicate		
contemplate		
complacent		
automobile		
negligence		

More Practice Words

Syllable Identification	Number of Syllables	Stress Patterns
quadruple		
recorder		
underprivileged		
appendages		
apprehend		
advertisement		
ambivalent		
vivacious		
development		
diversify		
environment		
indecision		
atmosphere		
spirituality		
pneumonia		
nonviolence		
tolerance		
spontaneous		
satisfaction		
professional		

Adopting Weaker Articulation

Deletions

Instructions: Review the list of /h/ deletions in "he"/"her." Then write the "deleted" form used in each of the practice sentences. Then practice reading the sentence out loud.

did he   = **did'e**

didn't he = **didn'e**

will her   = **will'er**

did her   = **did'er**

  1. (Did he) leave you a key to his suite?

  2. (Did he) want me to call him a cab?

  3. How (did he) get home?

  4. Where (did he) leave the report for me?

  5. (Didn't he) get my message?

  6. (Didn't he) return your books on time?

  7. Why (didn't he) finance this project?

  8. Why (didn't he) leave early for the airport?

  9. Where (will her) new office be?

10. When (will her) promotion be authorized?

11. Why (will her) husband do that?

12. (Will her) surgery be scheduled for today?

13. (Did her) vacation request get approved?

14. When (did her) contract end?

15. How (did her) signature get on this document?

16. (Did her) colleagues accept the apology?

17. (Did he) share his success with you?

18. (Didn't he) have the same problem last time?

19. What (will her) boss say when he sees the report?

20. (Did her) car get towed?

Deletions in "have" Helping Verbs

Review the list of "have" helping verb deletions. Then write the "deleted" form used in each of the practice sentences. Then practice reading the sentence out loud.

could have = could'uv	couldn't have = couldn'uv
would have = would'uv	wouldn't have = wouldn'uv
should have = should'uv	shouldn't have = shouldn'uv
must have = must'uv	mustn't have = mustn'uv

1. I (could have) taken the bus.
2. They (could have) waited longer.
3. Without your seatbelt, you (could have) been killed!
4. She (could have) asked me for a ride.
5. It (couldn't have) been that cheap.
6. She (couldn't have) called me two days earlier because she was sick.
7. Without your help, this plan (couldn't have) been successful.
8. Hong Kong (couldn't have) been as cold as Madrid!
9. You (would have) been proud of me today!
10. If I had known earlier, I (would have) helped out.
11. She (would have) reached home by now, I suppose.
12. I (would have) preferred something hot, actually!
13. I (wouldn't have) resigned from this job if I knew about the merger.
14. If you hadn't told me, I (wouldn't have) known about it at all!
15. This was one time that she wouldn't have) refused to help out.
16. If I know Susan, she (wouldn't have) left the front door open.
17. Knowing the weather forecast, they (should have) left for the airport by noon.
18. The physician (should have) ordered x-ray studies sooner to rule out a fracture.
19. I (should have) done a better job in planning this party.
20. It's been four weeks—her arm (should have) healed.
21. Mrs. Brown (shouldn't have) missed her class.
22. She (shouldn't have) waited till the last day to turn in her paper.
23. I (shouldn't have) tried to do everything myself.
24. My boss (shouldn't have) authorized the fund raiser.
25. Someone (must have) left the phone off the hook.
26. I (must have) misunderstood your comment about the promotion.
27. This (must have) been a complete shock for your family.
28. Diane (must have) contacted a lawyer about her divorce by now.
29. You (mustn't have) closed the door yesterday afternoon.
30. The team (mustn't have) detected the problem during the initial inspection.

Add-ons

Instructions: Review the /h/ words, such as "he," "her," "his," "hers," when followed by "is," and listen for the change heard in rapid speech. Practice saying the words in parentheses in the sentences that follow. Then practice reading the sentence out loud.

is he	= **iz'e**
isn't he	= **izn'e**
is her	= **iz'er**
isn't her	= **izn'er**
is his	= **iz'iz**
isn't his	= **izn'iz**

1. (Is he) going to pull out your tooth this week?
2. (Is he) going to the conference on emotional trauma in August?
3. He's not the current president of the company, (is he)?
4. (Is he) really going to run the Boston Marathon next year?
5. (Isn't he) going to Alaska for a vacation next week?
6. Josh is a great motivational speaker, (isn't he)?
7. The boss is on vacation and Kyle is acting as the manager, (isn't he)?
8. He *is* going to sign this contract, (isn't he)?
9. (Is his) wife still working at the framing shop?
10. (Is his) report on the project almost ready?
11. John has lost weight, but (is his) blood pressure under control?
12. (Is he) here alone or (is his) daughter with him?
13. (Isn't his) balance paid as of the end of the month?
14. That (isn't his) project to criticize.
15. Why (isn't his) performance evaluation on my desk?
16. Why (isn't his) boss at this important meeting?
17. (Is her) company making any profits?
18. I hope that this (is her) last project for this quarter.
19. Where (is her) case file on the new client?
20. (Is her) house on the market?
21. Why (isn't her) boss accompanying her to this meeting?
22. Tuesday (isn't her) birthday.
23. (Isn't her) son in the army?
24. That (isn't her) problem.
25. (Is he) ready for this new project?
26. (Is her) mother helping her plan the wedding?

27. (Isn't her) her job too stressful right now?

28. (Isn't he) the one who groomed John for the promotion?

29. (Is his) sister going to retire soon?

30. (Isn't his) buddy, Shane, a manager at Systems, Inc.?

"You" Add-on

Instructions: Review the following list of "you" add-ons. Then work through the practice sentences, reading each one aloud. The IPA transcription is provided for the first sentence in each grouping.

do you	= **do yə**
will you	= **will yə**
don't you	= **don' tʃu**
didn't you	= **didn' tʃu**
did you	= **did dʒu**
had you	= **had dʒu**

1. (Do you) like writing short stories or fiction?

2. (Do you) mind watching the kids for me?

3. How (do you) manage to juggle work and home?

4. You don't want a time out, (do you)?

5. Where (do you) go for lab work?

6. (Will you) be going to the party on the fifth of September?

7. What (will you) do after you retire?

8. Who (will you) pick for your project?

9. You won't be tired after all that dancing, (will you)?

10. How (will you) make it back on time?

11. (Don't you) find New York City interesting?

12. You do remember the initial training, (don't you)?

13. What (don't you) like about the project format?

14. Why (don't you) like this proposal?

15. I find her fascinating, (don't you)?

16. You did mail that important package, (didn't you)?

17. Who (didn't you) include in your last memo?

18. You did accept your promotion, (didn't you)?

19. Why (didn't you) call the recruiter?

20. (Didn't you) know that the Dogwood Festival was being held this weekend?

21. Why (won't you) reply to your cousin's letter?

22. Who (won't you) invite to your graduation party?

23. What kind of promotion (won't you) accept?

24. You will be at the staff meeting, (won't you)?

25. Won't you be an angel and bring me the paper?

26. You had spoken to her about the report, (hadn't you)?

27. Who (hadn't you) called about the conference?

28. You had saved the whole document, (hadn't you)?

29. Why (hadn't you) told him about the doctor's visit?

30. (Hadn't you) mentioned that idea before?

31. You should be back in two days, (shouldn't you)?

32. What (shouldn't you) repeat to Ed?

33. Who (shouldn't be) invite to this meeting?

34. Why (shouldn't you) report this incident?

35. (Shouldn't you) be studying for your quiz?

36. (Wouldn't you) like to talk to him?

37. Where (wouldn't you) consent for a transfer?

38. Who (wouldn't you) like as the new director?

39. You would like to have the service, (wouldn't you)?

40. Why (wouldn't you) invite him to your graduation?

41. You could still drive, (couldn't you)?

42. Why (couldn't you) set timelines for this proposal?

43. When (couldn't you) call for the seminar?

44. Who (couldn't you) assign the project to?

45. (Couldn't you) have cleaned your room before everyone showed up?

46. When (did you) schedule the interview?

47. How (did you) achieve the projected goals?

48. You didn't ask for reassignment, (did you)?

49. Where (did you) buy your sweater?

50. (Did you) do as Mrs. Brown asked?

51. When (had you) worked with Margo in London?

52. I (had you) in mind for that promotion.

53. You hadn't given your resignation letter yet, (had you)?

54. Whom (had you) contacted in Cairo?

55. (Had you) contacted her before?

56. When (would you) like to see the house?

57. You wouldn't like to be treated that way, (would you)?

58. Whom (would you) call for assistance?

59. Why (would you) want to sell the stocks now?

60. (Would you) like to go to the show with us?

61. When (should you) be finished with your proposal?

62. You shouldn't add so much salt, (should you)?

63. How (should you) report this altercation?

64. Why (should you) buy it when you can get it for free?

65. (Should you) be playing a video game during homework?

66. How (could you) just leave the party?

67. When (could you) meet with the team?

68. Whom (could you) ask for a favor?

69. You couldn't wrap up the meeting by five, (could you)?

70. (Could you) tell me where the board room is?

Assimilation

Instructions: Say each of the practice sentences aloud, listening carefully for the assimilation. Then write the assimilated pronunciation and underline the letters involved.

Anticipatory Assimilation

Practice these assimilations in isolation before proceeding to the sentences that follow.

coin bowl = coi<u>m</u> <u>b</u>owl	good gimmick = goo<u>g</u> <u>g</u>immick
ten bibs = te<u>m</u> <u>b</u>ibs	good guy = goo<u>g</u> <u>g</u>uy
ten beats = te<u>m</u> <u>b</u>eats	good kite = goo<u>g</u> <u>k</u>ite
ten pleats = te<u>m</u> <u>p</u>leats	good game = goo<u>g</u> <u>g</u>ame
ten bites = te<u>m</u> <u>b</u>ites	good gum = goo<u>g</u> <u>g</u>um

1. Can I drop my change in your coin bowl?

2. The sales department came up with a good gimmick for the new product.

3. Do you really need ten bibs with every meal?

4. Your friend Sam is a good guy.

5. She was practicing at ten beats per minute.

6. That's a good kite to fly on a day like this.

7. Would you like ten pleats on your skirt?

9. It was a good game this weekend.

9. Take ten bites and finish your meal.

10. Wrigley's spearmint is good gum.

Progressive Assimilation

Practice these assimilations in isolation before proceeding to the sentences that follow.

that boulder (t>p)   that game (t>k)
that bum   that guard
that pipe   that glass
that bottle   that gum
that class   that gaper

1. That boulder is very heavy to lift, even with ten people.
2. She could have played better at that game.
3. That bum decided to drink too much at his friend's party.
4. Can you ask that guard for directions?
5. That pipe seems to be leaking.
6. That glass is half full.
7. Can I keep that bottle?
8. Stop chewing that gum!
9. Are you sure that class is at 7?
10. Are you finished with that paper?

Reciprocal Assimilation

Practice these assimilations in isolation before proceeding to the sentences that follow.

this sheep   his sharp tongue
this ship   this shoddy job
this sheet   this shape
this shampoo   this sharing
this shiny coin   this shipping

1. This sheep needs to be sheared.
2. His sharp tongue can do a lot of damage.
3. His favorite toy is this ship.
4. Who is responsible for this shoddy job?
5. Please make corrections on this sheet only.
6. This shape will do just fine on stage for a rock.
7. Who makes this shampoo?
8. This sharing stuff between roommates is getting out of hand.
9. This shiny coin belongs to . . .
10. This shipping company is filing for bankruptcy.

Exact Assimilation

Practice these assimilations in isolation before proceeding to the sentences that follow.

crepe paper	test tube
mad dog	sad day
fake coin	backed down
gag gift	what time
like Kyle	this sack

1. Do you have some crepe paper for this craft?
2. Where are the test tubes stored?
3. That mad dog lives in my neighborhood!
4. What a sad day it turned out to be.
5. Is that a fake coin?
6. After a lot of convincing, he finally backed down.
7. What was the gag gift at her party?
8. What time are we meeting the Jones?
9. Do you want to play soccer like Kyle?
10. This sack is full of rocks from our travels.

Connector Assimilation

Practice these assimilations in isolation before proceeding to the sentences that follow.

an éclair = a neclair	I'm up = I' mup
an ache = a nache	thumbs up = thum zup
an aide = a naide	mean act = mea nact
calm us = cal mus	an actor = a nactor
an apron = a napron	I'm ending = I' mending

1. I'm eating an éclair.
2. Okay, okay, I'm up.
3. She has an ache in her shoulder.
4. Thumbs up for a job well done.
5. What is the job of an aide?
6. That goes down as a mean act in my book.
7. Did she just say that to calm us down?
8. To be an actor is hard work.
9. I would like to sew an apron.
10. After this project, I'm ending my contract with them.

Other Variations Affecting Pronunciation

Suffix "-ed" Endings

Final t (or te) plus /əd/	Final d (or de) plus /əd/	Voiceless /t/	Voiced /d/	Voiceless /t/	Voiced /d/
tested	added	talked	paled	staffed	trained
frosted	padded	walked	spied	stuffed	strained
potted	shredded	stalked	tied	fluffed	stunned
toasted	threaded	parked	flowed	puffed	gunned
posted	sided	barked	bellowed	miffed	donned
busted	coded	marked	blamed	changed	chained
crusted	nodded	stacked	tamed	managed	stained
assisted	molded	worked	shamed	snipped	abstained
existed	decided	stroked	named	quipped	stemmed
melted	collided	poked	mimed	tripped	stoned
estimated	needed	processed	mooed	touched	snarled
devastated	degraded	stressed	booed	stretched	stirred
persisted	upgraded	pressed	judged	watched	barred
stimulated	glided	dressed	scaled	starched	stared
limited	confided	crossed	scowled	parched	sparred
commuted	up sided	splashed	ragged	scooped	deployed
promoted	down sided	trashed	jagged	hoped	stayed
connoted	kneaded	slashed	tagged	cooped	preyed
rotated	traded	crashed	wagged	looped	frayed
propagated	stranded	blushed	sagged	stooped	employed
retreated	concluded	tarnished	wedged	shipwrecked	restrained
re-enacted	compounded	banished	slogged	unmarked	preoccupied
emancipated	applauded	vanished	fogged	embarked	snorkeled
necessitated	commanded	finished	flogged	disembarked	buckled
resuscitated	surrounded	famished	mugged	remarked	positioned
substantiated	decoded	crushed	lugged	reworked	propositioned

Medial /t/ Sound as in "bitten"

Practice saying the words aloud. Review the IPA transcriptions for the first several entries. Then provide IPA transcriptions for the remaining entries.

English Spelling	IPA Transcription—within Conversation
Latin	Lætn = Latn
rotten	rɑtn = rottn
smitten	smɪtn = smittn
beaten	bɨtn = beatn
written	rɪtn = rittn
forgotten	fʌrgɑtn = forgottn
heighten	haɪtn = heigtn
unbeaten	ʌnbɨtn = unbeatn
typewritten	taɪpritn = typewrittn
flatten	
frighten	
enlighten	
rewritten	
sweeten	
mutton	
glutton	
brighten	
threaten	
lighten	
cotton	
tighten	
straighten	
fatten	
mitten	
Hutton	
gotten	

Medial /t/ Sound as in "water"

Practice saying the words aloud. Review the IPA transcriptions for the first several entries. Then provide IPA transcriptions for the remaining entries.

English Spelling	IPA Transcription—within Conversation
better	bɛtɚ = bɛdɚ
betting	bɛtŋ = bɛddŋ
data	deta = deda
heater	hɪtɚ = hɪdɚ
settle	sɛtl = sɛdl
suitor	sutɚ = sudɚ
total	totl = todl
notice	notis = nodis
sweating	
swatter	
rattle	
pretty	
flutter	
splutter	
platter	
beater	
bitter	
batter	
kettle	
metal	
nitty-gritty	
splitting	
blotting	
bunting	
mutter	

The Schwa (x) Factor

Practice saying the words aloud. Then provide the IPA transcription for each.

English Spelling	IPA	English Spelling	IPA	English Spelling	IPA
tool		feel		poor	
stool		seal		pure	
cool		squeal		sure	
school		McNeil		allure	
spool		O'Neal		obscure	

Silent e

Make sentences using each word in each pair. Then practice saying them aloud.

wag/wage	whack/wake	win/wine
stag/stage	tack/take	din/dine
rag/rage	snack/snake	fin/fine
sag/sage	lack/lake	dim/dime
hag/Hague	rack/rake	Tim/time

Final "-ous" /ʌs/ Pronunciation

Say the words aloud. Generate your own list of "-ous" words. Then provide the IPA transcription for each.

Final "-ous" Words	IPA	Your List of Final "-ous" Words	IPA
famous			
cautious			
gorgeous			
hilarious			
adventurous			
curious			
malicious			
suspicious			
capricious			
delicious			

12

Conversation: Strategies for Success

Your mastery of the basics and some of the idiosyncrasies of English paves the way to a higher level of fluency in speaking your new language. Now you feel ready to reap the benefits of what you've learned, converse easily and comfortably in your interactions with others. But especially as a speaker of English as a second language (ESL), you may find that conversations do not always proceed as expected. Miscommunication can occur even between native speakers of the same language, so various conversational mishaps are possible. No matter how much we hope for an "ideal" conversation, outcomes cannot be predicted.

This chapter introduces the protocols of good conversation. An important ingredient of conversation is a natural flow of discourse among the participants. Various strategies help to make the exchange of ideas and opinions, thoughts and feelings, smooth and easy to comprehend. In particular, conversational repair strategies can be used to maintain or restore this flow. The Suggested Reading section at the end of the book lists resources for additional information on how to hone your conversational skills.

Definition of Conversation

To define *conversation*, let's begin by distinguishing between dialogue and conversation. A *dialogue* is a conversational exchange between two people. For all second language learners, dialogues are worth all the effort of practice. Because the exchange of messages is between only two people, you will have better control of how you convey your message.

When there are more people involved in a conversation, however, steering the discussion toward where you want it to go becomes difficult. In addition, if you are shy, it becomes a challenge to interject your opinion on the subject of discussion. Using different simulated situations with appropriate vocabulary can make practice time educational. The rewards come later when all of your efforts lead to real communication.

The important thing to remember is that ideal conversation is a simple exchange of thoughts and feelings. It is *not* a powerful exposition of intelligence or wit, and it definitely is not speech making. It is a process of give and take that requires an ability to listen and to express interest in the other person while presenting one's own ideas and opinions politely, clearly, and meaningfully. Conversation can be between two or more people, so *dialogue* and *conversation* may sometimes be used interchangeably.

Is the art of conversation inherited? Or can the skills of conversation be mastered by hard work? Some people with infectious personalities make good communicators by mixing intellectual charm and wit—whereas others less gifted must apply themselves with the help of books, audio tapes, videos, or seminars to better their conversational skills. These differences exist among persons of all language backgrounds. But conversational skills are worth mastering because they will serve you well wherever the social and professional ladder takes you. With a high level of motivation and a deep desire to excel, you *can* become proficient in the art of conversation.

Components of a Good Conversation

What makes good conversations happen? For each of the components of conversation, certain general protocols are recognized.

Greetings

Whatever your country of origin, greetings will form the first part of any conversation. Every language has a set of phrases used exclusively for greetings. For people living in English-speaking countries, greetings generally are divided into social and professional greetings:

- *Social greetings* set the tone of the meeting, party, or family gathering. Informal, familiarly spoken greetings ("Hi!" "Hey, Buddy!" "Wow—look

at you!") may be accompanied by a handshake or a hug, depending on the relationship between the people greeting each other.

- *Professional greetings* are more formal and may or may not involve a handshake. The speaker may begin by saying "Hi!" or "Hello" or "How are you? My name is . . . " Then the conversation may turn immediately to business, with "Let's get started" or "Let's begin the meeting" or "What's on the agenda?"

Introduction of Topic

After the exchange of greetings, you will probably introduce a topic relevant to your relationship to the person(s) involved in the conversation (for the purposes of this discussion, let's assume you're the one taking the lead in the conversation). Selection of the topic is easier if the other person is a family member or friend. It is harder when the other person is just an acquaintance or, worse, someone you would rather avoid. A few general guidelines follow:

- "Formal" or specific topic introduction is necessary in professional conversations, meetings, or presentations. "Please refer to the agenda. We are going to start with . . . "

- Topic introduction is definitely more subtle in casual, social conversations, in which the talk typically flows smoothly from one topic to the next without anyone having to stop and pointedly introduce another.

- Different openings to conversations may include but are not limited to asking for directions, recipes, or advice or opinion about restaurants, sports, politics, preparing for a party, and so on.

- Giving compliments is a good way to open a topic of conversation. End the compliment with an open-ended question so that you do not get short or one-word responses. For example: "I heard you did a great job organizing the holiday party at the office. What was the hardest part in coordinating it?"

- If you are already aware of the person's hobbies, sports craze, or even a few likes or dislikes, you may use any of this information as an opening topic to lend a personal touch. If you prefer to keep the topic general, however, weather, sports, and politics are good stand-bys.

Continuity of Conversation or Topic Manipulation

Conversations occur in such a way that topics can be continuously introduced, sustained, altered, and reused. As a second language learner, you will gradually learn how to manipulate the topic in conversation as your language and vocabulary systems develop and your vocabulary bank of cultural slang and idioms expands.

There are various ways to keep the conversation flowing. If you are unsure of what to say, prepare ahead of time by rehearsing your vocabulary. Here are a few suggestions:

- Humor is the best way to keep a conversation pleasant and enjoyable. Witty comments, using idiomatic expressions, amusing stories, and socially appropriate jokes, add "flavor" to an ordinary conversation.

- Vary the sentence formats used to exchange ideas and convey your message; choose from among statements, questions, requests, and exclamations. If you listen critically, you will notice that all of these sentence formats are used repeatedly during any conversation.

- Linking related topics using "Wh" questions (where, what, why, when) or "How" questions helps to keep the continuity of conversation.

- Open-ended questions are better than closed-ended questions. Questions that elicit a yes-or-no answer or "thank you" may be regarded as closed-ended questions. Open-ended questions elicit responses that elaborate or explain in some detail, in contrast with a single-word response. The following are examples of open-ended questions: "How was your trip to Hawaii?" "Tell me about your trip to Hawaii." "What is the status of your project report?" "What is your opinion on the (topic)?"

- Comments or questions that elicit controversial responses should be avoided in order to maintain a pleasant tone within the conversation. Unless a meeting was prearranged to address controversial issues, for example, statements of conflict are best avoided.

- Compliments can be used to create a positive tone in initiating or continuing any conversation. You can compliment the person's abilities, recent accomplishments, apparel, and so on.

- It also is necessary to learn how to receive compliments. Here are a few statements to use in rehearsing how to accept compliments.

  1. "Thanks—I had to work hard to organize it." [*You did a great job organizing the meeting.*]

2. "I am glad you like it. I was lucky to find it at that antiques dealer in town." [*I love your grandfather clock.*]

3. "It's nice of you to say so—I made it myself." [*I love your sweater.*]

4. "Thanks for noticing. It was pretty difficult coordinating everything." [*You put in a lot of effort—the band, the seven-course meal—for this party.*]

New Topic Insertion

Nobody likes awkward silences in conversations. It then becomes necessary to quickly and smoothly introduce a new topic. Any of several different techniques can be used.

- You can make comments that lead into another topic. For example, let's say the initial topic of conversation with a friend is the weather. After a few conversational turns, you may subtly switch to talking about rainy weather gear, which is a new topic but related to the initial topic.

- You can introduce an entirely new topic: "Did you know what happened last week?" "I forgot to tell you that I can't make it to your party next week." "Before I forget, let me remind you that we have our regular book club meeting this month." "I don't mean to be rude, but I would like to say something about that." Such statements politely but firmly divert the conversation away from the original topic.

- New topics also may be introduced according to the likes and dislikes of the friend or family member. With acquaintances and strangers,

however, sticking with general topics of weather or sports, for example, is always safe and polite.

Listening

Key to effective and successful conversation is listening attentively. It conveys your respect for and interest in the speaker—and also is the hallmark of a good conversationalist. You will be able to respond appropriately to the speaker's questions and comments only if you practice good listening. In addition, listening to yourself speak helps you monitor when your turn ends and another's turn begins. If necessary, refer back to Chapter 8, on auditory discrimination, to review critical listening.

Turn Taking

It is vital to monitor yourself as you speak because you need to recognize when to let the other person have a turn in the conversation. If only one person is talking, the "conversation" is not even a dialogue—it's only a monologue or, worse, a speech or a lecture.

You also need to know when it is acceptable for you to "break in" for your turn to speak. What are the turn-taking indicators in a conversation?

- Pay attention to when the speaker is pausing, which may indicate that you can have a turn to speak without seeming like you are rudely interrupting.

- Pay attention to intonation variations in stress patterns that signal the end of the sentence (as discussed in Chapter 9, on intonation).

- Use phrases such as "I'd like to say something about that . . . " or "I would like to add . . . " or "I think that . . . " to signal that you are ready to take your turn.

- Conversation clarifiers such as "What I meant to say is . . ." or "Let me rephrase that . . ." or "Maybe I should have said it another way . . ." or "If I had to say it again . . ." also can be used to signal your turn.

- Listen for the use of conversation starters and clarifiers by other people in the group, as such phrases indicate their readiness to take their turn.

Nonverbal Communication

Nonverbal communication is an important indicator in turn taking and management of any conversation. Body language conveys feelings and attitudes and makes a lasting impression, sometimes even before words are spoken. Use of nonverbal communication in conjunction with speech is very common and enhances understanding of any spoken language. The superiority of visual representation for communication is well recognized, as indicated by phrases such as "Every picture tells a story" and "A picture is worth a thousand words"; likewise, body language can be a dead giveaway of the speaker's feelings and attitudes. If necessary, refer to Chapter Ten to review how nonverbal communication influences conversation.

Eye Contact

Although eye contact is addressed in Chapter 10, it is worth mentioning again because it is the most important indicator within a conversation. Eye contact signifies rapt attention on the speaker and is essential to the success of all types of conversations. Any wavering of eye contact is interpreted as inattention, boredom, and evasiveness. Eye contact thus conveys the listener's interest or lack of interest in either the speaker or the subject matter. So for the interaction to be successful, proper eye contact is essential throughout the conversation.

Interruptions

According to the dictionary, *interrupt* means to cut short, disrupt, butt in, or barge in—all somewhat negative connotations. And people often do interrupt in a negative manner. Then the dialogue changes from a simple conversation to an animated discussion or maybe even an argument. There are different ways, positive and negative, to respond to such interruptions.

- In a gathering of family or friends, when some one interrupts or speaks out of turn, use of casual phrases to reclaim the role of speaker such as "Hey, wait a minute—I was still talking" or "May I finish talking, please?" is customary and acceptable.

- A person who is frustrated or annoyed may respond with "Don't keep interrupting me" or "I am not finished yet" or "I am not done talking" or "Don't butt in!"

Interruption of another person during conversation is occasionally acceptable, however, and there are a number of socially acceptable phrases used for this purpose. In such cases, the interruption is perceived as polite interjection.

How do you make interruption acceptable? A few appropriate phrases include the following;

- "Excuse me for interrupting."
- "May I say something?"
- "Pardon me, but I have a question . . ."
- "I would like to add to that comment."
- "I would like to make a comment."

Sometimes in a large group situation (meetings, classrooms), raising your hand to attract the attention of the speaker in order to make a comment also is acceptable.

Concluding or Terminating a Conversation

Terminating a conversation can be considered an art, especially for a non-native speaker. It is considered rude to abruptly leave without indicating that the conversation is finished. Here are some ways to accomplish tactful conclusion of your conversation.

- *Professional meetings*: To conclude a meeting, a formal "wrap-up" is essential. The presenter probably is following an agenda and will make a reference to it at the appropriate time. The speaker will clearly indicate that the conference is finished by saying "Meeting adjourned" or with a simple "Thank you for attending this seminar."

- *Important social gatherings*: With weddings, anniversary parties, company Christmas parties, and so on, a formal goodbye is expected. It is considered polite to seek out the host family, compliment them on their entertaining skills, and thank them for their hospitality.

- In other conversations, you can politely excuse yourself by saying, "Please excuse me—I am in a hurry" or "I'm running late—sorry, I have to leave" or "Pardon me— I am in a rush."

- Between family and friends, conversation endings are more casual; "I have to go, Mom." "I guess I'd better let you do your work—bye." "I have to go pick up my son from daycare—see you

later." "I am in the middle of . . . , so I'd better get back to it."

- You probably are familiar with the following concluding or final phrases: "Bye!" "See you later." "Have a nice day." "Have a nice evening/night." "Goodnight!"

To summarize, a successful conversation depends on the following:

- Utilizing all of the components of conversation

- Introductions and opening small talk

- Effective question/answer techniques—asking and responding appropriately

- Inclusive behavior—through eye contact, turn taking

- Understanding and responding to invitations—inviting, accepting, declining, offering, declining, making arrangements

- Complimenting, showing appreciation

- Offering opinions, comments

- Farewells and reinforcing contacts

Refer to the worksheet at the end of the chapter for practice with different scenarios of conversation.

Survival Conversation Guidelines

Now let's take a look at some ideas you can use to survive conversation blunders. The Suggested Reading section lists a few excellent books for more detailed study.

Survival Do's of Conversation

Although you are beginning to use English as a main vehicle for communication, you still may be somewhat unsure of usage and vocabulary, especially idioms. So a list of the "do's" of conversation is provided to help you simplify all of the components of conversation into a natural, easy interaction. Once you master these simple guidelines, you will find it easy to apply them within your conversation.

- Do provide information only if you have evidence to back it up.
- Do present the message with genuine pleasantness.
- Do establish and maintain eye contact throughout the interaction.
- Do practice appropriate turn taking to include everyone in the group.
- Do speak only as much as necessary.
- Do keep the message "short and sweet."
- Do use simple, short words versus lengthy, compound words.
- Do pay attention to the time and conclude the conversation appropriately.
- Do use vocabulary words only if you are sure of their usage.
- Do keep the content of your speech relevant to the topic.
- Do provide additional details only if requested.

Enroll in a "Vocabulary Workout Program"

Vocabulary is an integral part of any conversation. To have a conversation, you need to have the words. Memorizing vocabulary lists is tedious, however. Nevertheless, vocabulary usage in everyday communication is always being tested, because adults are not in the habit of formal study to increase their vocabulary. Keep in mind, however,

that sincere effort and self-motivation to increase your vocabulary bank will enhance the clarity and presentation of your speech. Here are a few tips to improve your vocabulary.

- Start with new words of known structure or similar word groupings (at, hat, bat, cat, and so on).
- Substitute new words in sentences of known word pattern (He has a cat/rat).
- Change sentence patterns with the same vocabulary words (Cats are good pets/Dogs are good pets).
- Use grammatical markers such as tense or number (singular versus plural) to make word lists (act, acts, acted, acting; smile,, smiles, smiled, smiling).
- Sort words into related categories to increase your word list (fruits, furniture, countries, places of worship, places of work, things that move, things that are square, things that are brown, and so on).
- Develop categories within categories to generate a vocabulary tree (public places/post office/stamps/ letters/cover letters/memos, and so on).
- Learn new words through participation in professional or social organizations and events and use them consistently.
- Write down all new words identified within everyday conversation and use them in different sentences.

Use of a Direct Approach

Within conversations, speech that is clear and concise usually is considered most effective and is appreciated by others. Being direct (but not rude) and to the point is an excellent survival guideline to remember at all times.

- State what you mean and request what you want. Do not "beat around the bush" (i.e., don't ramble on) because this indirect approach can allow others to make incorrect assumptions, potentially leading to misunderstanding.

- If you or another person doesn't have the information needed: Within casual communication, responses such as "I'll try and get that information for you" or "I'll call you back with the phone number/information" or "I'm not sure, but I can find out" usually are acceptable.

- In business communication, a more specific response is necessary: "I will verify and have the answer to you by 3 PM."

Use of "Punctuation" within Conversation

Most ESL speakers initially find it hard to organize their thoughts and stay on topic within the conversation. There's a temptation to present an impression that they know the language very well, with lots of vocabulary words, so they speak at a rapid pace to "get all the words in."

If you were writing down what you say, you would use punctuation marks such as periods and commas to indicate a pause or a break in thought. But within spoken language or conversation, you use the intonation patterns of stress and pauses (as described in Chapter 9 on intonation).

So when you are speaking, it is natural to pause and take a breath where your sentences end (which could be with a period or a question mark or even an exclamation point), instead of rambling on so that all the words seem to run together without a break. Indications that you are not pausing appropriately include requests for clarification from the listener: "Wait a minute—can you go slower and repeat that?" "Say that again, please." "I am not sure I understand what you said." (Refer to the section on pauses in Chapter 9.)

You also can request clarification from American speakers. As a non-native speaker of English, you may find the average American's "normal" pace of speech to be too fast for you. Don't be shy about asking for clarification—such requests indicate to the speaker that you are being attentive and are sincere in wanting to fully understand the message that is being conveyed.

Use of Fillers or Conversation Connectors

What do the following comments have in common?

- "Let me think."
- "Give me a second here."
- "It's like this . . . "
- "Let me explain."
- "Don't you agree?"
- "Well . . . "
- "Uh . . . "

These are all "fillers"—words or phrases that "fill up" the time it takes to process information received in conversation and then respond. Instead of allowing awkward silences to develop, a majority of people use fillers in most casual conversation. In professional situations, use of fillers is considered offensive and annoying. Bert Decker, a communication specialist, refers to fillers as "non-words." He considers them to be barriers to clear communication if they are used frequently. However, an occasional usage within the natural flow of conversation may be acceptable.

Fillers have acquired their poor reputation because as single words or short phrases, they are easy to overuse, often to the point of annoyance to the listener; furthermore, they force the listener to wait until "real" information is provided. But in my experience, sometimes brief sentences, carefully worded to engage the listener, can be very useful to tie in new information to the topic of discussion, to provide thinking time, or to fill up the time needed for the person to respond appropriately. For such sentences, interjected within the course of a conversational turn, I prefer the term *conversation connectors* instead.

Conversation connectors not only connect or link thoughts between conversational turns but also allow for clarifications, explanations, and comfort. They provide comfort to both the speaker and the listener by setting aside enough time to receive the information, process it, and respond to the messages conveyed. Unless the interaction is a debate, conversation connectors reassure the participants that conversation is a medium to express thoughts and feelings respectfully and meaningfully, and not a powerful demonstration of brainpower or wit.

For example, let's say you are posed with a somewhat difficult question and you need a few minutes to get your thoughts together. It is not perceived as wrong to say "Let me think for a moment and I'll get back to you" *or* "I'll have the answer for you at the end of this lesson." You may have heard public speakers or your teachers or professors use these particular conversation connectors.

Here is a list of highly effective conversation connectors compiled from my own years of listening to skilled speakers at seminars;

- "So what you're saying is that . . . "
- "There are several different ways to answer that question."
- "Enough said on that topic. Moving right along . . . "
- "I am telling you this in confidence, but . . . "
- "I'm sorry—I misunderstood your remark."
- "I'm sorry that I was unaware of your problem."
- "I apologize—I completely misread your comment."
- "Let's try to figure this out together."
- "I need to think about it first."
- "I have a point to add."
- "I would restate what she said as . . . "
- "I am not sure where this topic is headed, but . . . "
- "Let's get back to the main topic."

Nevertheless, communication with almost no "non-word" fillers, appropriate pausing, and an extensive vocabulary is the desired standard for clear and lucid communication. Most foreign-born persons tend to use their native language fillers while learning English, which adds to the confusion of the listener. If you are a non-native speaker of English, you must become aware of such fillers within your native language and how they affect your speech in the new language. In addition, you must familiarize yourself with the conversation connectors of the English language to increase your expertise in all interactions.

Although we have been using the term "conversation connectors," speech-language researchers from early on have used the term "conversational repair strategies" to describe what people do for clarification and correction of messages in conversation. These approaches assist both speakers and listeners to have a successful interaction. The strategies have the following functions:

- Allow for modification or correction of your message
- Allow to rephrase or repeat requests for clarification
- Allow for indication of misunderstanding
- Allow requests for details or expansion

These are exactly the functions of our conversation connectors! Whether you call them fillers, conversation connectors, or repair strategies, they are crucial for a successful interaction. In the natural flow of conversation in any language, everyone unconsciously uses these strategies or their cultural variations. Evidently, everyone acquires these strategies by trial and error beginning in childhood. As you grow older, you develop the ability to use these strategies in various communication interactions. Some people master the skills of repair so well that they become masters at manipulating any situation, social or business.

Use of Contextual Cues

You are already aware that every conversation starts out with an initial topic. And ongoing conversation uses vocabulary and language related to that topic. It is important that you never assume that everyone uses language in same way as you. Therefore, if the message is somewhat confusing, use the context or your general knowledge of the topic to verify information.

In addition, to determine the exact meaning of a message, it often is helpful to consider a few other factors: who is saying it, how it is being said, when it is said, where it is said, and why it is being said. Making a request for clarification using conversation connectors is far preferable to misunderstanding the message or remaining misinformed.

Survival Vocabulary and Language

Personal Remarks or Comments

What's the correct response if someone makes an unkind remark to you, or disparages an ethnic group or nationality during a conversation with you or in a group discussion? In such cases, your first instinct probably is to get angry. This makes communicating your thoughts very difficult. It is much harder to speak clearly and convey your meaning effectively, even in your own language, when you are upset.

And for non-native speakers of English, responding under stress is even more difficult. Not responding at all, even though you are upset, could be one course of action. Another would be to respond with an angry retort—and if the ESL speaker happened to use wrong words that turned into an inappropriate comment, a total misunderstanding could result, leaving you frustrated and unable to defend the comment.

Rehearsing some common phrases or sentences for general situations, therefore, is not a bad idea. Here's a list of such statements you can put away in your vocabulary bank for later use if the need arises.

- "I don't appreciate your comment."
- "Let's change the topic."
- "Let's get off this subject."
- "I wish you had something nice to say instead."

- "Don't you think that remark was uncalled for?"
- "Why would you want to make a mean remark like that?"
- "I'm sorry—that remark was insensitive."
- "I'm sorry—that remark was tasteless."
- "I wish you had stated that comment more positively."
- "I'd like to know why you don't agree with me."
- "I'm surprised at the rudeness of that remark."

Tact and Tactlessness

Frequently, personal remarks and tactlessness go together. According to Webster's dictionary, *tact* is a keen sense of what to do or say in order to avoid conflict and to maintain good relations with others. Applying tact can avoid assumptions and inferences that lead to miscommunications and misunderstanding among friends, family members, and co-workers.

Here are a few examples of questions and statements that are less than tactful or are even in poor taste.

- "What's the matter with your child?" (question asked in a critical tone and posed to the parent of a mentally impaired child)
- "Are you and Tom really getting a divorce?"
- "I heard from your neighbor that you are pregnant. Congratulations!" (Wait until the person tells you she is pregnant before congratulating her, so you know for sure, instead of finding out that it was false information or that she has lost the pregnancy.)

- "What did you pay for your house/ car?" [or any other financially related topic] (If you feel uncomfortable responding, try one of these responses to deflect the question: "I don't remember what it cost. Why do you want to know?" "I can give you websites that my agent gave us to get comparables in your area." "I'd rather not talk about it. With the cost of living being what it is, the whole subject is discouraging.")

Telephone Etiquette

When you call someone on the telephone, it is important to identify yourself first and then ask to speak to the person. For example: "This is Kim. May I speak with Mrs. Smith?" Accents are very hard to decipher over the phone. Because the caller's face is not visible to the person called, the usual cues from reading facial expressions and interpreting mouth movements are not available to help in clarifying the message. Especially during phone conversations, it is essential to stress the important words to get your message across.

Other Foreigners, Other Accents: Mixing and Mingling to Support Conversational Skills

You are not alone in your experience of conversational mishaps as an ESL speaker. Other immigrants also encounter such mishaps and, just like you, continually seek various ways of eliminating these embarrassing moments. Increasing your awareness of accents of other non-native English speakers to identify similarities and differences will help create an atmosphere of support for one another in your common quest for conversational knowledge.

Mingling with other immigrants will help ease the feelings of isolation from others due to your accented English. In addition, you can compare your accent and language usage with those in other non-native English speech you hear, to identify any similarities and differences. If you associate only with other immigrants who speak your native language, you will not be able to keep from reverting to use of that language and you will forget to practice English.

For example, in an English conversation class I taught, several students were Hispanic, but from different countries—Spain, Columbia, Peru, and Puerto Rico. Each of them spoke a dialect of Spanish. During the 2-hour class, they tried their best to speak only English, lapsing into Spanish only if translations and explanations were not adequate. As soon as they left the classroom, however, they reverted back to Spanish, because the ease of conversation in their native language was just too tempting.

In another class, however, the students consisted of only one native Spanish speaker and others whose native languages were Korean, Indian, Chinese, and French. Because they did not know each other's language, they had to maintain conversation only in English, with no opportunities to revert back to their respective native languages. All of these students made much better progress because of the benefit of conversing with only English speakers, even though the English they all heard was mostly non-native English.

Summary

Now that you know that conversation has its own protocols, you can apply the techniques and strategies presented in this chapter to help make each of your conversational interactions as meaningful or enjoyable as possible. We all expect to have an ideal conversation every time we start or join one, but it helps to remember that outcomes of conversation cannot be predicted. Most people are aware of the components and rules of conversation—yet conversational mishaps still occur. With such mishaps, it is the responsibility of each of us as a participating conversationalist to use the appropriate repair strategies to smooth things over.

The following thoughts from experts on social discourse and the art of conversation are worth keeping in mind:

If you aspire to be a good conversationalist, be an attentive listener. To be interesting, be interested. Ask questions that the other person will enjoy answering.

—*Dale Carnegie*

"I" is the smallest letter in the alphabet. Don't make it the largest word in your vocabulary.

—*Dorothy Sarnoff*

In a conversation, instead of saying "I think . . . ," ask: "what do you think?"

—*Socrates*

WORKSHEET 12

Conversational Skills Activities

Instructions:

- Audio taping dialogues for realistic feedback can help you with self-awareness in all aspects of conversation and accent management.

- Practice free dialogue/conversation using a predetermined topic with family, friends, or even cooperative colleagues.

- Review the components and rules of conversation and apply them when practicing the following exercises.

- Rehearse appropriate dialogue for each of the example scenarios so that you will be more prepared for real-life situations as they arise.

1. Role play
    - cashier/customer
    - pharmacist/customer
    - stewardess/passenger
    - doctor/patient
    - nurse/patient
    - supervisor/employee
    - babysitter/employer

2. Telephone activities
    - making an appointment
    - ordering take-out from a restaurant
    - asking and giving directions
    - enrolling a child in school
    - finding information about a product or for buying a car or a house
    - interviewing

3. Face-to-face activities
    - asking for information at the library
    - opening a bank account
    - parent-teacher conference
    - bargaining a price
    - ordering food at a restaurant

- interviewing
- speaking up at meetings

4. Situations requiring greater tact/conversational skill
   - speaking with your boss or manager
   - offering condolences at a funeral
   - returning an item to the store
   - lodging a complaint
   - participating in a conference workshop

5. Successful socializing: Use the following examples to rehearse and hone your conversational skills

Introductions:

- "Hi, my name is Sally Hansen. How are you?"
- "This is John. He is new to our group."
- "We haven't met. I'm Susan. I work with Sally."
- "Let me introduce to two communication specialists, Ms. Maya Brown and Ms. Eva Rain."
- "Here comes my favorite person—Joseph Dean."

Question/answer techniques:

- Making requests

  Scenario 1

  "May I have a drink please?" *or* "Can I offer you something to drink?"
  "Sure thing."
  "What kind would you like—alcohol or soda?"
  "I prefer diet soda, thanks."
  "Do you not drink alcohol for religious reasons?"
  "Not really. I just choose not to drink alcohol."

  Scenario 2

  "Can I ask you a favor?"
  "Try me."
  "Can I borrow your snow blower this weekend?"
  "Absolutely."
  "Thank you. I appreciate it."

- Declining
  "No, thank you."
  "Maybe later."
  "Water is fine, thanks."

- Understanding and responding to invitations
    1. Inviting
        a. "I would like to invite you to my daughter's graduation party. Can you come?"
        b. "Would you like to come to my summer get-together?"
    2. Accepting
        a. "Yes, we would love to be there."
        b. "Sure—we wouldn't miss it for anything!"
        c. "Of course! How can I say no to my best friend!"
        d. "Sounds like fun. I will be there."
    3. Declining
        a. "I'm sorry—I have to decline your invitation, as I've got a previous commitment."
        b. "I may have to take a rain check this time."
        c. "I have other plans that weekend. Maybe next time!"
    4. Making arrangements
        a. "Do you need help setting up for the party?"
        b. "Is there anything I can do to help you?"

Complimenting, showing appreciation:

- "Excellent work. A job well done."
- "What a beautiful sweater you have on. Did you knit that yourself?"
- "I am so grateful for all your help. Thank you."
- "You did a great job planning this wedding.
- "You took your responsibility seriously and completed the task on time. It's admirable!"
- "This agency does outstanding work."
- "Jo, you came up with a brilliant idea."
- "Thanks to Sandy's tremendous effort, the company has developed a first-rate product."

Offering opinions, comments:

- "May I say something?"
- "I would like to say one thing in support of . . . "
- "My view on this issue is . . . "
- "If I may counter that argument . . . "
- "My comment here is . . . "
- "This is what I think . . . "
- "In my opinion, it means . . . "
- "The fact of the matter is . . . And that's my opinion."

Apologizing:

- "I'm sorry for . . . " *or* "I apologize for . . . "
Potential reasons:
bad behavior
lack of punctuality
missing a party/event
not being helpful when needed
misunderstanding and clearing up

Offering condolences:

- "I am sorry to hear about your . . . "
Potential reasons:
losing a job, promotion
losing a family member or friend
illness/injury to a family member or a friends

Farewells and reinforcing contacts:

- "Pleased to have met you. Let's stay in touch."
- "Here is my number. Call me when you're in my neck of the woods. Bye."
- "See you later, I hope."
- "Maybe we should meet for dinner later in the week to discuss your idea."
- "Maybe we should get together sometime."
- "I had such a great time. We should do this again."

6. Paraphrasing

- For excellent vocabulary practice, try *paraphrasing*—rephrasing written material to present the same information. You can use either more or fewer words or sentences for your rephrasing.

- Use short articles from magazines or newspaper to begin your practice. With longer articles, choose two or three paragraphs to work with at first and gradually progress to include the whole article.

- Rephrase descriptive passages by recapping a recent event, for example, or summarizing an informational article. Here are a couple of "articles" to start with.

Vegetarian Style

Like many people living in America, you may eat vegetarian meals all or part of the time. But just because a dish is vegetarian doesn't always mean it is healthy. You still have to watch out for hidden calories from carbohydrates, which break down into sugar, and from fat in the oils used in cooking the vegetarian dish. You also need to pay attention to the method of cooking—roasting, grilling, simmering, or lightly stir-frying, versus deep-frying—which could affect your weight and health.

Most people who are trying to adopt a vegetarian diet assume that the choice of foods is less, so they perceive this way of eating as "boring." But you can get lots of variety by trying foods from other countries. International cuisine is gaining in popularity. People are not only dining in various ethnic restaurants but also trying their expertise in cooking ethnic dishes at home. With the opening of many international grocery stores and the availability of many of the ingredients in your local supermarket, it's easy to experiment with ethnic food preparation in the comfort of your own home, to adjust the seasonings to your taste. Keep in mind that using low-fat or nonfat ingredients and making the right choices at restaurants will help to achieve a healthy vegetarian lifestyle.

The Story of Language

For centuries, people all over the world have wondered about the origin of language. How did words come to exist? How did they come to be combined to make sentences and develop into a language? Do all languages have a single source? These questions are fascinating and have been posed repeatedly by each generation in futile attempts to find the answers.

Linguists and scientists all over the world are conducting research and experiments only to reach the same dead end: lack of evidence. Researchers have gone to extraordinary lengths but are hampered by the vast and distant time scale involved. We have no direct data of the beginnings and early development of language. Moreover, it is very difficult to imagine how such knowledge could ever be obtained.

Therefore, researchers will continue to speculate, arrive at conclusions, and remain somewhat dissatisfied—or be inspired to delve deeper into its mysteries to find more. We do know for a fact that this research is ongoing, so the "story of language" has yet to be told in full.

Conclusion: Some Final Thoughts . . . and a Look Ahead

Now you have embraced a new approach to accent modification, incorporating not only multiple, highly effective strategies but also an appreciation of the ties of language to culture, the wonderful utility of the phonetic scripts, and the music of intonation. You've had a glimpse into the scope of practice of speech-language pathology to help you decide whether to get some professional coaching in foreign accent management—or as a possible career path for yourself!

The concept of foreign accent management presented in this book is based on a combination of valuable techniques with practical ideas, compiled from published research and my own participation as a professional in workshops, tutoring sessions, and speech therapy, as well as my personal experiences as an ESL learner. Several of the techniques described for different aspects of the foreign accent management program have been in practice in one form or another for many years and were devised orig-

inally by researchers in the fields of speech-language pathology and linguistics.

In this book, a "pure" linguistics perspective, with a detailed analysis of similarities and differences between languages and their effect on accents, has been avoided, for the sake of simplicity and a reader-friendly format. Ongoing research by phoneticians and linguists, however, will continue to deepen our literature stockpile regarding the mysteries of all language and accents. When you are ready to dig deeper, refer to the "Suggested Reading" section for some excellent selections to help you continue your journey with foreign accent management.

The basic methods used in foreign accent management are tracking the error sounds and applying strategies and techniques of correction. Over time, you will grow more comfortable with use of these skills. With your new skills emerging, you will detect an increase in your level of comfort in speaking English. Besides figuring out the commonalities between immigrant customs and languages, you also will learn to monitor the effects of your native language on your accent.

As you sharpen your skills, your accent will change for the better or may even be erased. Once you have mastered how to manipulate your articulators through use of these indispensable techniques, you can learn to "switch" between accents. For a brief but formal business presentation, for example, you may consciously switch from native language—accented English to "genuine" American English—and then back again for a casual conversation with friends who are used to your "accented" speech. (You may even go to the extent of imitating your own accent before someone else does it to ridicule you!) This flexibility means that you can control and manage your accent in all manner of business and social situations, building your confidence and greatly curtailing the possibility for those embarrassing moments.

Here are some general principles you can use in your approach to foreign accent management:

- Apply the techniques and strategies to one issue at a time. You will learn to deal with your issues more assertively and be able to take on new accent challenges confidently.

- Evaluate yourself periodically to see where you stand. Ask a friend or a trusted colleague to assess the difference in your speech since you started working on your foreign accent management. You may able to self-correct your speech most of time, but the view of a third person is always valuable.

- Keep in mind that complete generalization of your new speech patterns in all types of situations and conversational circumstances takes time to achieve. Accordingly, patience and persistence are the key.

Although you've reached the end of this book, you also are beginning a long relationship with the practice of foreign accent management and cultural communication. Difficulties and challenges will continue to arise, but with hard work you can achieve great progress in improving your spoken English and creating an attractive accent. This should give your confidence and self-esteem a wonderful boost!

Feel free to write or e-mail me (at mythri_fam2000@yahoo.com) with questions, comments, or ideas at any time. You will be contributing to my stockpile of real-life experiences that I can use to teach more immigrants like you and me.

Postscript:
Musings of an Immigrant

It's easy to forget that most people living in the United States are either immigrants or descendants of immigrants. Only Native American Indians are truly "native" to this country. But today we are beginning to imagine *all* of the citizens of the world as brothers and sisters, with English being the common connection, the thread that binds us together. Living together is necessarily a process of give and take, an exchange of culture and customs, while we enjoy the similarities and appreciate the differences.

Whether out of respect for our own immigrant ancestors or out of empathy with other ESL learners, each of us can reach out a helping hand to the newcomers who have come to live in or visit this land of opportunity. By taking on the role of a teacher, you will be helping the novice immigrant settle in with ease and dignity. And by playing the role of ambassador of your native country, you may be relieving fears of "otherness" and increasing tolerance of differences, unlocking the doors to a whole new world of cross-cultural communication.

Most important, we all need to remember that we did not wish for or choose our native language and customs. We were born into or inherited these cultural characteristics. And although we don't want to lose them in the process of trying to "fit in," acceptance into a new and different community is crucial. Nevertheless, preserving the beauty of your culture and richness of your language and accent is equally important, as it is a deep and essential part of who you are. You can change your hair color, for example, to purple or another extreme hue not found in nature, or to the exact opposite of your own, whether it's the darkest black or the lightest blond—but underneath you will still be the "natural" version of yourself. In adapting to a new culture, it's important to work on finding a balance between who you have been and who you are becoming, to let the truest you emerge.

My education in language, accent, and culture began when I set foot on American soil. The "coursework" has been challenging, and I do not see a final exam coming up any time soon, to settle my competence once and for all. Instead, my foreign accent management program has become a permanent "work in progress." Every time I've conquered an accent demon, another one crops up! I finally realized that there is always more to discover, more to learn—making my accent-cultural learning an ongoing endeavor.

One of my goals as an ESL speaker is to create a near-perfect American English accent in my speech while continuing to absorb the cultural and linguistic idiosyncrasies, no matter how long it takes. My rationale is that if my host country is making an effort to understand different cultures and accents, it seems only fair to do my part to fit in with colleagues and friends. Another goal is to retain some flavor of my "Indian-accented English," to maintain my roots and an appreciation of my culture and customs—and pass on this heritage to my daughter and other generations to come.

Although native speakers of American English can and will continue to detect the mishaps in my vocabulary and accent, "putting on" an American accent has so far been successful professionally and socially for me. It is my belief that when we open pathways of communication with people of diverse cultures and languages, our own insights are sharpened. This is exactly what has happened during my work with accent management. Discovering the similarities in the culture and customs—"Hey, we do that too!"—has made it exciting. The recognition that "they" are not so different after all—that there is no "us" and "them"—has been a pleasant eye-opener. Learning about the variations has allowed me to expand my cultural horizons and has increased my own levels of tolerance. The final revelation has been that the "accent on acceptance" and the "dialect of compassion" are the same in all languages!

Glossary

Accent
A characteristic of pronunciation that is natural in every person's speech and is indicative of his or her geographical origin.

Articulation
A process or an act of speaking using the articulators (vocal organs) to produce speech sounds in specific patterns and combinations to make meaningful words.

Articulators
The vocal organs—structures of the mouth and upper portion of the throat, including specific muscles, used to produce speech. Also see *Oral-motor*.

Auditory discrimination
The ability to distinguish speech sound differences between and within words (e.g., /cap/ versus /cab/).

Body language
A manner of using gestures, facial expressions, and posture to communicate emotions and feelings during a conversational exchange.

Conversation
A verbal exchange of thoughts and ideas between people.

Consonants
The letters denoting speech sounds produced by vocal tract obstruction of air flow shaped by the specific placement of the articulators.

Dialect
An offshoot of a language that usually sounds similar to the original language but has unique differences that distinguish it from the original language.

ESL (English as a second language)
Describing a non-native speaker of English —a foreigner whose first language at birth is not English but who is learning to speak English; also used to describe courses taken by ESL speakers.

Homonyms
Words that are spelled alike but are pronounced differently (e.g., *tear* from the eye, *tear* in a dress).

Homophones
Words that sound alike but are spelled differently (e.g., *right, write, rite. Wright*).

International Phonetic Alphabet (IPA)
A set of symbols that depict the speech sounds of the English language, used by linguists and speech-language pathologists.

Intonation
The music or melody of language that attaches feelings and emotion to words and phrases to convey personal meaning.

Intonation, contrastive
The variation of intonation pattern that can be modulated or altered to emphasize

the exact meaning in the right context within any conversation.

Language
A set of sounds and symbols organized into combinations and patterns (words and sentences) used to communicate thoughts and feelings.

Linguist
A scientist who specializes in the study of various aspects of languages; a multilingual person.

Morphology
The study of how morphemes (the smallest meaningful unit of language) are combined to create words.

Non-native speaker
A person whose primary language—spoken in the country/region of the person's birth or rearing—is *not* the same as the language of the geographical region where he or she is residing currently.

Nonverbal
Referring to a method of communication that does not include oral language, or to use of gestures, expressions, and body language.

Oral-motor
Oral refers to the mouth and upper portion of the throat, encompassing the articulators. *Motor* refers to movements of these parts, which must to be precise to produce connected speech.

Phonemes
The speech sounds that are the basic units for word formation and are divided into vowel sounds and consonant sounds.

Phonetics
The study of phonemes, speech sound process analyses, and related topics.

Phonetic transcription
The process of writing words using IPA (see *International Phonetic Alphabet [IPA]*) symbols to denote the correct pronunciation of each word in any language, despite accent differences.

Pitch
The modulation or variation in tone of the speech signal or voice that provides a perceptual or auditory characteristic.

Script
Any of the alphabetic characters used in a language.

Semantics
The aspect of language that pertains to the meaning or description of the words.

Simulated (activity or exercise)
Referring to an activity that is made up for the purposes of learning or teaching.

Speech-language pathologist, speech therapist
A qualified professional in the field of speech-language pathology with specialized training in diagnosis and treatment of communication disorders and other language problems.

Stress
A manner of pronunciation within a word or word phrase used to demonstrate the importance of that syllable or word and to communicate the message strongly (to make a point).

Syllables
Units of spoken words that are larger than a segment but smaller than a word itself and made up of speech sounds in various combinations.

Syntax
The grammatical aspect of language that pertains to the rules and regulations that govern the process of forming words and combining into sentences; grammar.

Vocabulary
The stockpile of words that provides appropriate language and terminology for use

during conversations and other forms of verbal communication; a word bank.

Turn taking (in conversation)

To allow another person to take his or her chance at speaking or giving an opinion.

Vocal tract

The anatomic region consisting of the front of the mouth down to the throat that forms a pathway for the air to flow out from the lungs for the production of speech sounds; can be pictured as a hollow tube.

Vowels

The letters of the alphabet denoting the most important speech sounds for characterizing words; produced by altering the dimensions of the vocal tract to various degrees.

References and Suggested Reading

References

Adams, W. T. (1987). *Body English: A study of gestures.* Glenview, IL: Scott, Foresman and Company.

Blockcolsky, D. V. (1990). *Book of words: 17,0000 words selected by vowels and diphthong.* San Antonio, TX: Communication Skill Builders.

Blockcolsky, D. V., Frazer, M. J., & Frazer, H. D. (1979). *40,000 selected words. Organized by letter, sound and syllable.* San Antonio, TX: Communication Skill Builders.

Bernthal, J., & Bankson, N. (1981). *Articulation disorders.* Englewood Cliffs, NJ: Prentice Hall.

Colvin, J. R. (1997). *I speak English. A guide to teaching English to speakers of other languages.* Syracuse, NY: Literacy Volunteers of America.

Compton, J. A. (1992). *Phonetic transcription of foreign accent.* San Francisco: Carousel House/Institute of Language and Phonology.

Crystal, D. (1987). *The encyclopedia of language.* New York: Cambridge University Press.

Cummings, D. W. (1988). *American English spelling.* Baltimore: Johns Hopkins University Press.

Decker, B. (1997). *The art of communicating: Achieving interpersonal impact in business.* Menlo Park, CA: Crisp Publication.

Ehrilch, E., Flexner, B., Stuart, C. G., & Hawkins, M. J. (Eds.) (1980). *Oxford American dictionary.* Pleasantville, NY: Oxford University Press.

Eisenson, J. (1998). *How to speak American English.* Oceanside, CA: Academic Communication Associates.

Flowers, M. A. (1990). *The big book of sounds* (4th ed.). Austin, TX: Pro-ed.

Gangale, C. D. (1993). *The source for oral-facial exercises.* East Moline, IL: Lingui Systems.

Hall, E. T. (1992). *The hidden dimension.* Magnolia, MA: Peter Smith.

Hegde, M. N. (1985). *Treatment procedures in communicative disorders.* San Diego, CA: College Hill Press.

Johnson, J. (1980). *Nature and treatment of articulation disorders.* Springfield, IL: Charles C Thomas.

Lazzari, M., Peters, A., & Myers, P. (1987). *Handbook for exercises for language processing* (Help Series). East Moline, IL: Lingui Systems.

McAllister, L. (1994). *"I wish I had said that": How to talk your way out of trouble and into success.* New York: John Wiley & Sons.

Merriam-Webster's Collegiate Dictionary (10th ed.). (1999). Springfield, MA: Author.

Morris, D. W. H. (1988). *A dictionary of speech therapy.* London: Whurr.

Nicoll, L. (1993). *All work and no play: Social skills for business people.* Longman American Business English Skills series. London: Longman Group UK.

Nicolosi, L., Harryman, E., & Kresheck, J. (1989). *Terminology of communication disorders speech-language-hearing.* Baltimore: Williams and Wilkins.

Rosenbek, J. C. (1984). *Treating articulation Disorders: For clinicians by clinicians.* Baltimore: University Park Press.

Secord, W. (1981). *Eliciting sounds. Techniques for clinicians.* San Antonio, TX: The Psychological Corporation.

Sikorski, L. D. (1988). *Mastering effective English communication.* Santa Ana, CA: LDS & Associates.

Shewan, C. M., & Bandur, D. L. (1986). *Treatment of aphasia: A language-oriented approach.* San Diego, CA: College Hill Press.

Stefanakos, K., & Prater, R. (1982). *Auditory rehabilitation.* Austin, TX: Pro-Ed.

Westfall, M. (1998). *Greetings! Culture and speaking skills for intermediate students of English.* Ann Arbor, MI: The University of Michigan Press.

Suggested Reading

Althen, G. (1988). *American ways: A guide for foreigners in the United States.* Yarmouth, ME: Intercultural Press.

Burghart, J. (1990). *Living in the U.S.A. 2: A competency-based novel for intermediate students of English.* Lincolnwood, IL: National Textbook Company.

Calero, H. H. (2005). *The power of non-verbal communication: What you do is more than what you say.* Taking Control series. Lansdowne, PA: Silver Lake Publishing.

Gabor, D. (2001). *How to start a conversation and make friends* (rev. ed.). New York: Fireside Press/Simon & Schuster.

Garner, A. (1997). *Conversationally speaking: Tested new ways to increase personal and social effectiveness.* New York: McGraw-Hill.

Hinde, R. A. (1975). *Non-verbal communication* (New Ed ed.). New York: Cambridge University Press.

Lanier, R. A., & Davis, J. C. (2004). *Living in the U.S.A.* (6th ed.). Boston: Intercultural Press.

Martinet, J. (1992). *The art of mingling: Easy, proven techniques for mastering any room.* New York: St. Martin's Griffin.

Nierenberg, G. (1990). *How to read a person like a book.* New York: Pocket Books/Simon & Schuster.

Olayinka, J. (2006). *Turn your accent into an asset: How to deliver a dynamic speech even if English is not your first language.* Houston, TX: Indigo Riverbanks Books.

Shepard M. (2005). *The art of civilized conversation: A guide to expressing yourself with style and grace.* New York: Broadway Books.

Shiraev, E., & Boyd, G. L. (2000). *Accent of success: A practical guide for international students.* Englewood Cliffs, NJ: Prentice Hall.

Index

311

V

Vowels
as in "about" first vowel sound, 73–74
as in "all"/"call," 76–77
as in "baby," 88
as in "bat"/"thank," 67–68, 69–70
as in "beet," 87
as in "bet," 88
as in "bit," 87
as in "box," 72–73
as in "boy," 78–79
as in "calm," 70–71
cardinal system, 63
classification, 62–63
as in "coke," 75–76
diphthongs, 63, 78–82
IPA (International Phonetic Alphabet),
    33–35, 37–38
as in "out," 81–85
overview, 61–62
phonetic transcription, 43, 44
phonetic *versus* alphabetic sounds, 63
portrait/descriptions, 62–63
pronunciation, 63
"r-colored," 91–106
short and long sounds, 86–899

spelling, 63
as in "sun"/"but," 67–68
as in "time," 79–80
worksheets, 37–38

W

Worksheets
accent awareness exercises, 196–197
auditory discrimination, 204–212
consonants, 113–184
consonants, alphabetic/phonetic script,
    39–40
conversation skills, 295–299
intonation, 225–234
listening, 204–212
nonverbal awareness activities,
    247–248
oral-motor workout, 20–21
pronunciation, 267–282
questionnaire, communication/accent,
    11–12
vowels, alphabetic/phonetic script,
    37–38
vowel sounds, 66–106
World English, 187